Trauma and Emergency Surgery - The Role of Damage Control Surgery

Edited by Georgios Tsoulfas and Mohammad Meshkini

Published in London, United Kingdom

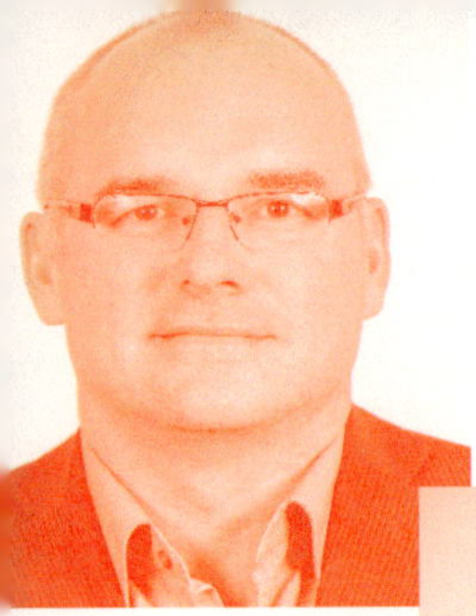
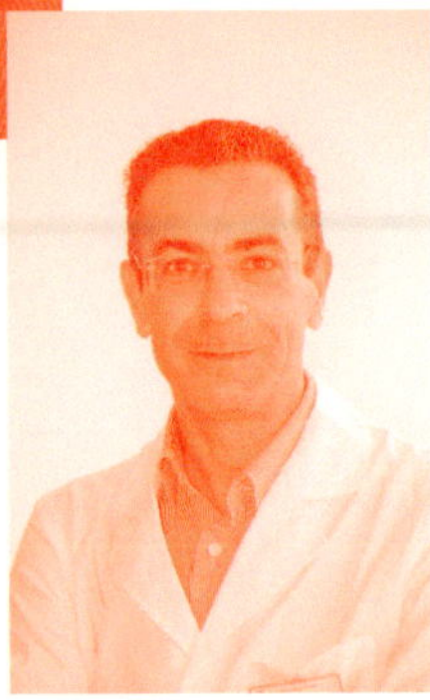
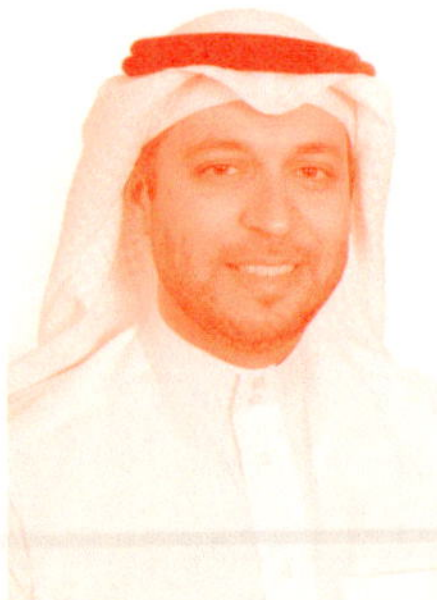
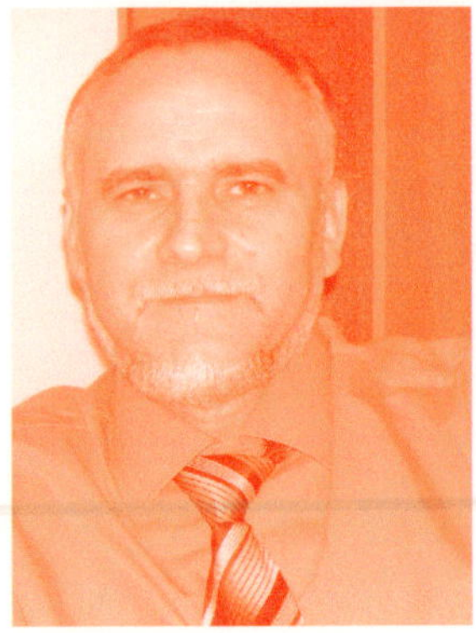
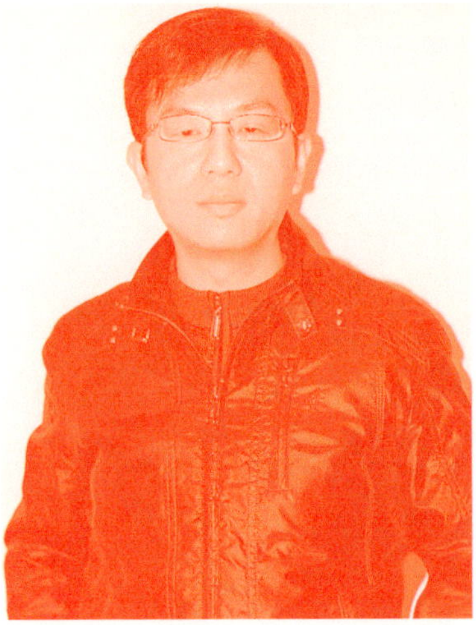
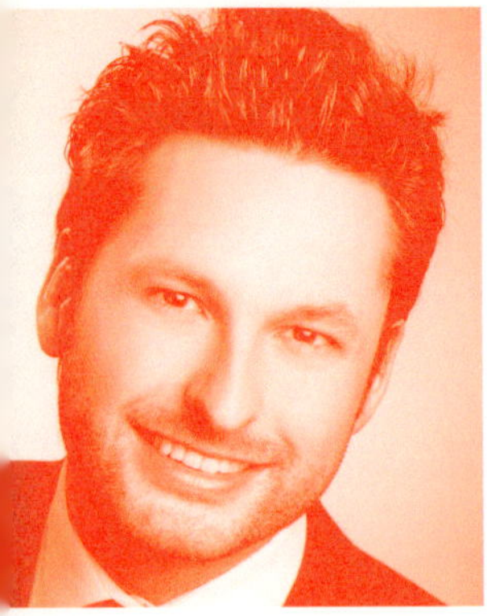
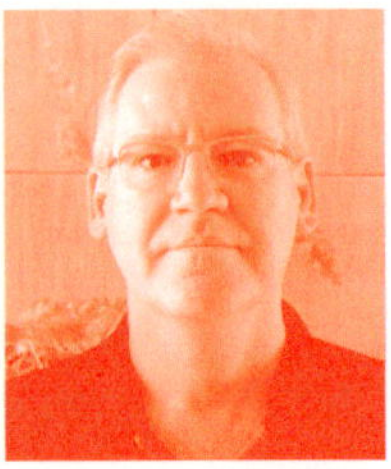

IntechOpen

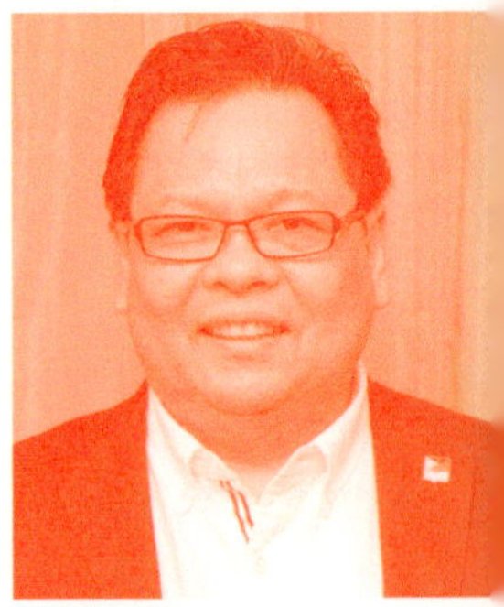
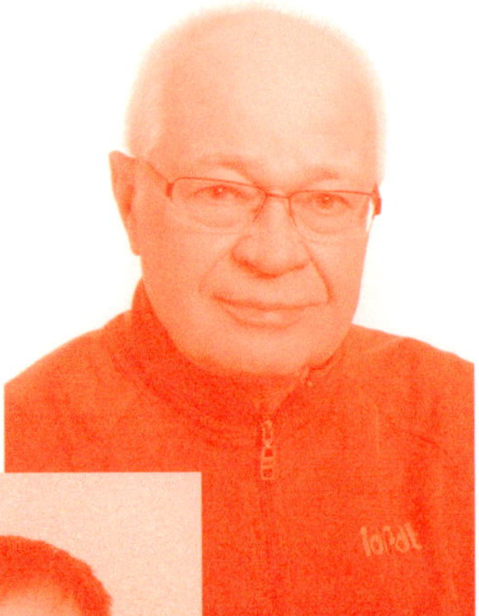
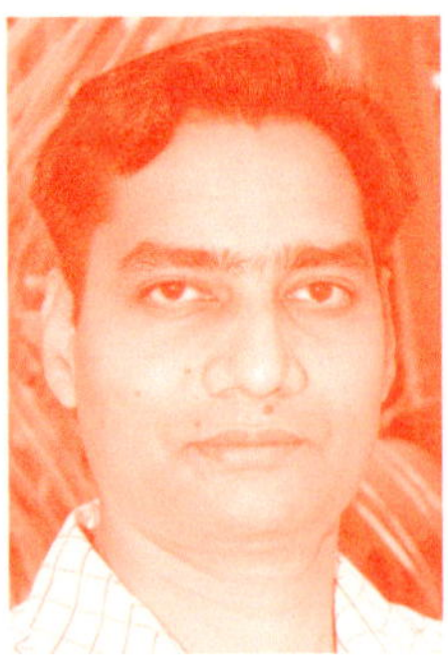
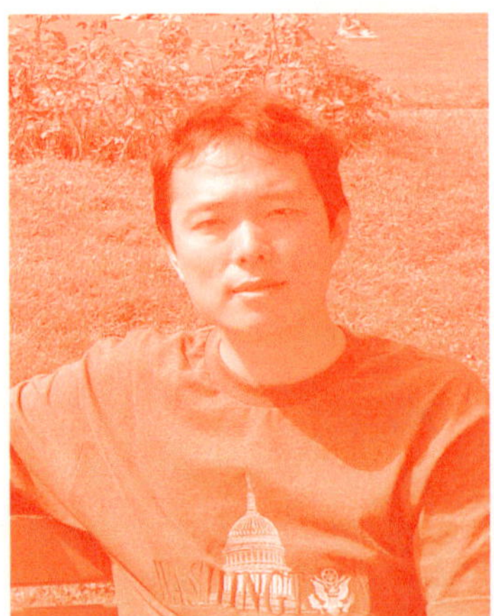
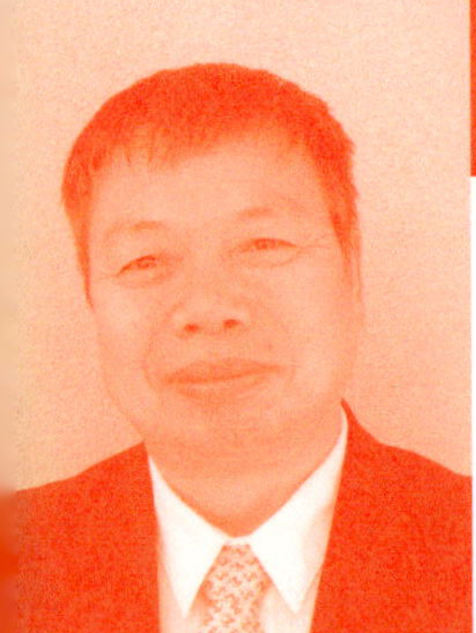
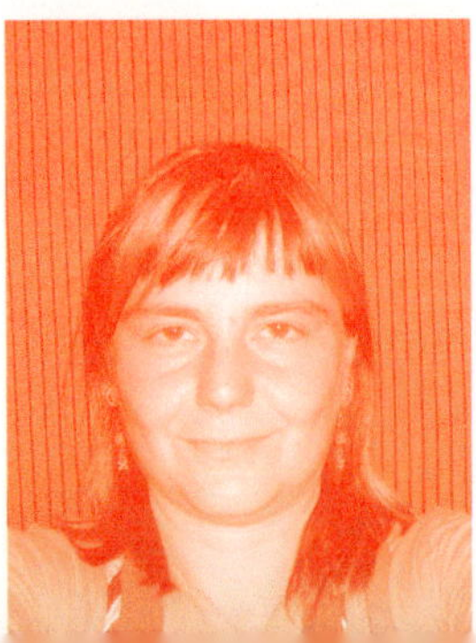

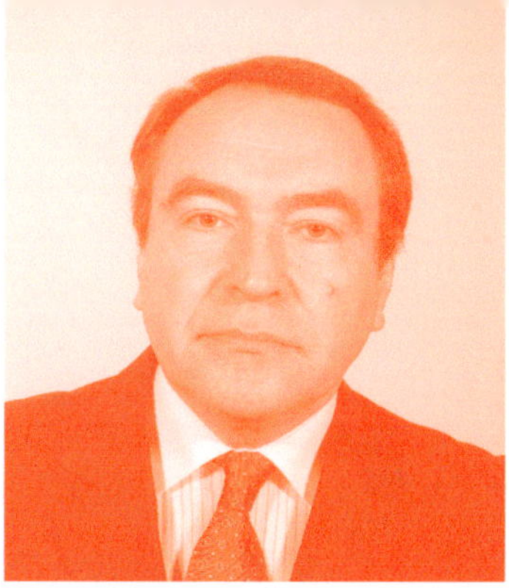

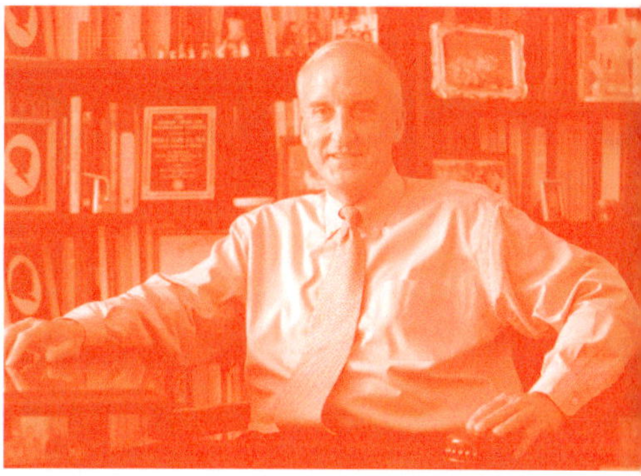

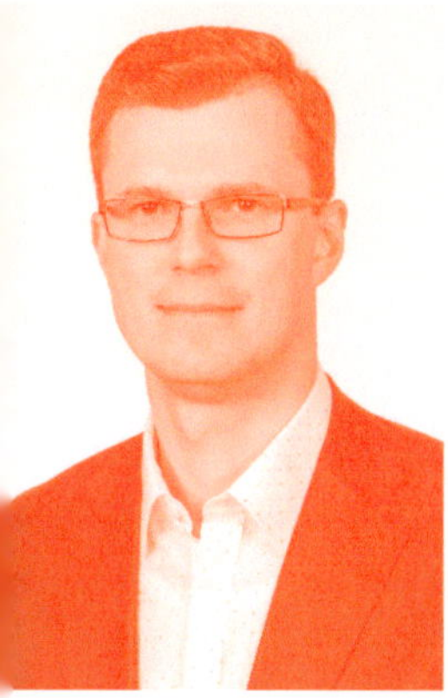

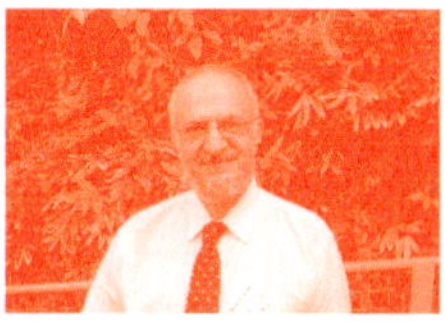

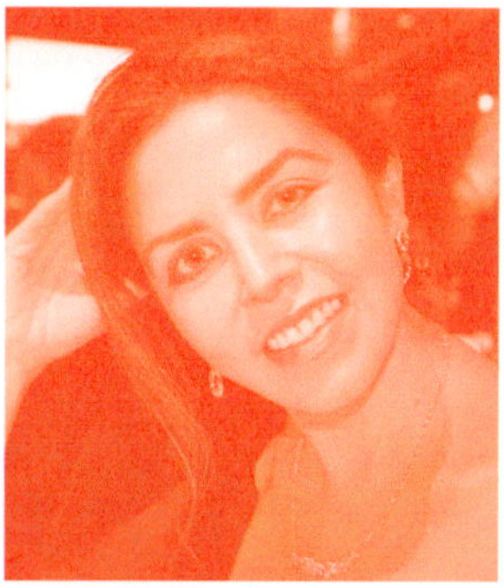

Supporting open minds since 2005

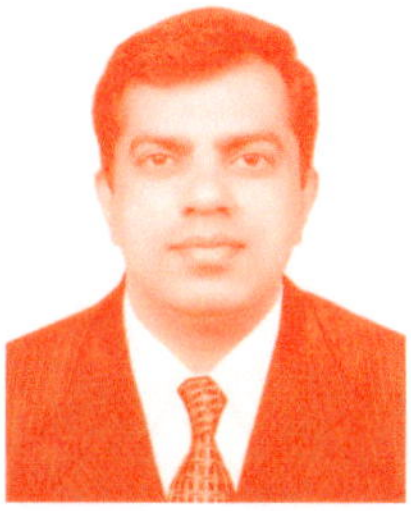

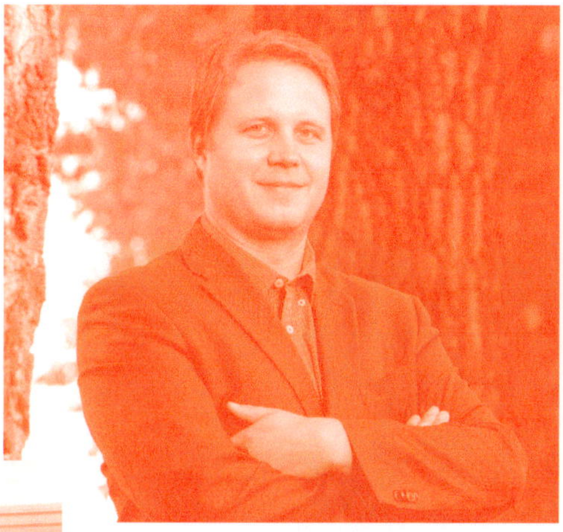

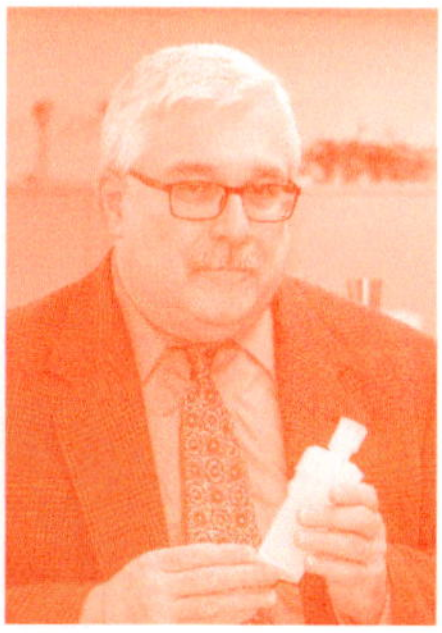

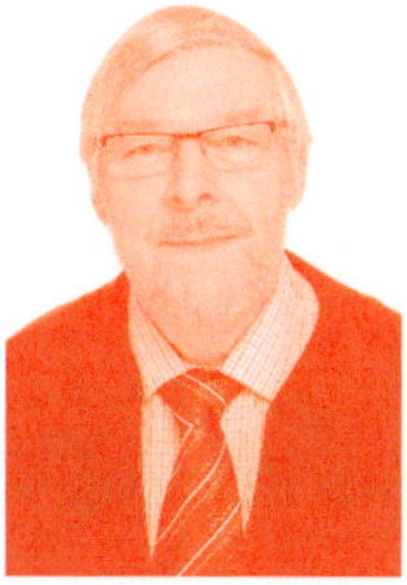

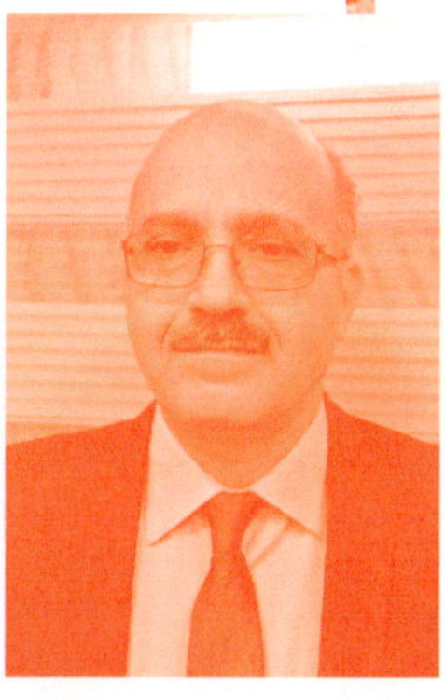

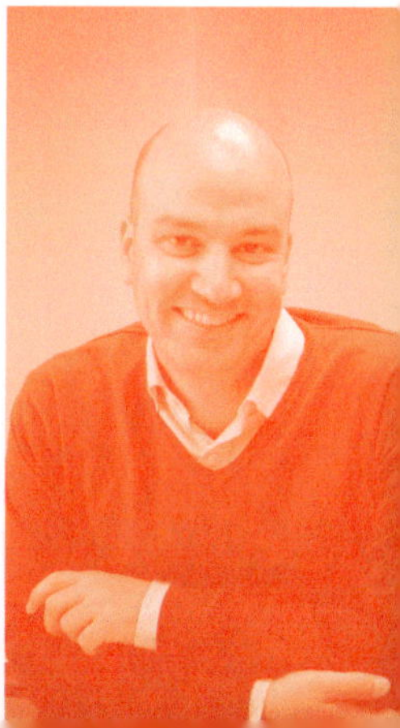

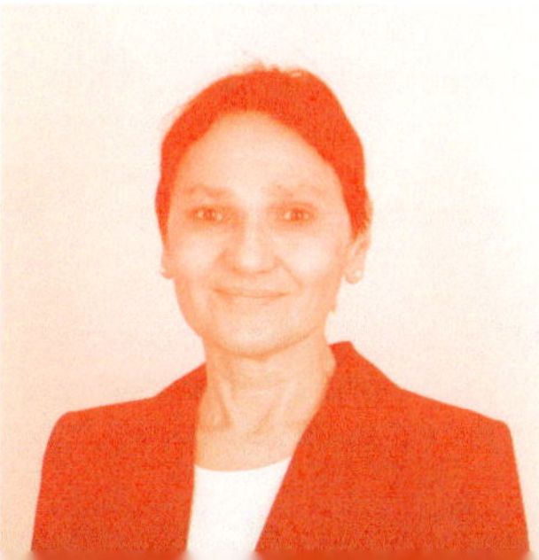

Trauma and Emergency Surgery - The Role of Damage Control Surgery
http://dx.doi.org/10.5772/intechopen.87629
Edited by Georgios Tsoulfas and Mohammad Meshkini

Contributors
Alfredo Alvarado, Yueh-Bih Tang, Shihheng Chen, Henrique A. Wiederkehr, Lucas M. Sarquis, Oona T. Daronch, Julio Cesar Wiederkehr, Barbara A. Wiederkehr, Lucas Scopel, Luca Ponchietti, Nestor Bueno Vidales, Andrea Casamassima, Fernando Gallego Estrada, Alessandro Garcea, Ioannis Gerogiannis, Alberto Lafita Lòpez, Diego Mariani, Olga Marin Casajus, Matteo Marconi, Nuno Filipe Muralha Antunes, Jorge Vera Bella, Carlos Yáñez Benítez, Pradal Jarne Laura María Pradal Jarne, Daniela Vrinceanu, Bogdan Banica, Mihai Dumitru, Georgios Tsoulfas, Ioannis Ziogas, Ioannis Katsaros, Marina Boushra, Thomas J. Fitzgerald, James Shen, Linda Ding, Kevin O'Connor, Ameer L. Elaimy, Carla Bradford, Fenghong Liu, Abdulnasser Khalifeh, Suhong Yu, Harry Bushe, Jonathan Saleeby, Kenneth Ulin, I-Lin Kuo, Yankhua Fan, Maryann Bishop-Jodoin, Paul Rava, João V. Zeni, Hung-Chi Chen

First published in London, United Kingdom, 2021 by IntechOpen
IntechOpen is the global imprint of INTECHOPEN LIMITED, registered in England and Wales, registration number: 11086078, 5 Princes Gate Court, London, SW7 2QJ, United Kingdom
Printed in Croatia

British Library Cataloguing-in-Publication Data
A catalogue record for this book is available from the British Library

Additional hard and PDF copies can be obtained from orders@intechopen.com

Trauma and Emergency Surgery - The Role of Damage Control Surgery
Edited by Georgios Tsoulfas and Mohammad Meshkini
p. cm.
Print ISBN 978-1-83968-164-6
Online ISBN 978-1-83968-165-3
eBook (PDF) ISBN 978-1-83968-166-0

For EU product safety concerns:
IN TECH d.o.o., Prolaz Marije Krucifikse Kozulić 3, 51000 Rijeka, Croatia, info@intechopen.com or visit our website at intechopen.com.

Meet the editors

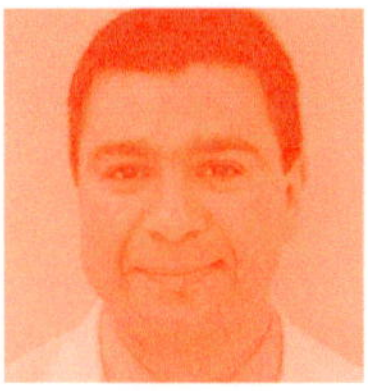

Dr. Georgios Tsoulfas received his medical degree from Brown University School of Medicine, Rhode Island, and completed his general surgery residency at the University of Iowa Hospitals and Clinics, as well as a transplant research fellowship at the Starzl Transplant Institute at the University of Pittsburgh. He then completed a two-year transplantation surgery fellowship at the Massachusetts General Hospital, Harvard Medical School, and then joined the Division of Solid Organ Transplantation and Hepatobiliary Surgery at the University of Rochester Medical Center as an Assistant Professor of Surgery. He has currently moved back to Greece, where he is an Associate Professor of Transplantation Surgery at the Aristotle University School of Medicine and Chief of the Transplantation Surgery Department in Thessaloniki, Greece. He has published more than 120 papers in peer-reviewed journals and in PubMed, as well as seventeen book chapters. He is a reviewer for more than forty international journals and on the editorial board of several others. He is currently Chair of the International Relations Committee of the American College of Surgeons and World President of the International College of Surgeons.

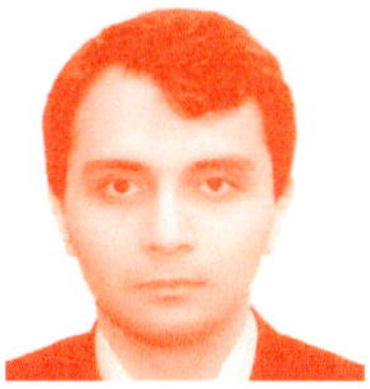

Mohammad Meshkini, MD, is an MPH candidate in his last year of a residency in Emergency Medicine at Iran University of Medical Sciences. He is an instructor candidate for courses in Basic Life Support (BLS) and Advanced Cardiovascular Life Support (ACLS) courses from the American Heart Association (AHA), as well as the Advanced Trauma Life Support (ATLS) course from the American College of Surgeons (ACS) and the Ultrasound Trauma Life Support (UTLS) course from the All India Institute of Medical Sciences (AIIMS). He has collaborated with the Iran Emergency Medical Services headquarters in Tehran, Iran. His fields of interest are traumatic patients and disaster management. Before choosing a career in emergency medicine, Dr. Meshkini pursued a Ph.D. in Disaster Healthcare Management.

Contents

Preface

One of the most interesting and challenging fields of medicine and surgery is trauma and emergency surgery. It is a continuously evolving field, as it incorporates the knowledge and skills of trauma surgery, emergency general surgery, and intensive care. The goal is to be able to approach these patients, who are in a life-and-death situation, in a more well-rounded manner.

A basic concept in trauma and emergency surgery is that of damage control surgery, as it provides surgeons with a strategy that allows them to prioritize the threats to the patient and manage them in a manner that shows appreciation of the physiology of the disease process, and not as simply a surgical exercise.

This book contains contributions from an excellent group of world authorities in the field of trauma and emergency surgery. In addition to the knowledge shared, the authors provide their personal clinical experience, making this book an extremely useful tool for every scientist and physician practicing in the field of trauma and emergency surgery. The book is divided into 3 sections with chapters showing the application of damage control surgery in different surgical specialties.

Overall, this book represents a true tour de force of a variety of topics having to do with trauma and emergency surgery. It should be stressed that the intended audience is scientists and physicians and surgeons of different specialties that all have in common an interest in trauma and emergency surgery and improving the lives of these patients.

Georgios Tsoulfas
Associate Professor of Transplantation Surgery,
Department of Transplantation Surgery,
Aristotle University School of Medicine,
Thessaloniki, Greece

Mohammad Meshkini
Tabriz University of Medical Sciences,
Tabriz, Iran

Section 1

General Concepts of Damage Control Surgery

Chapter 1

Radiation Injury and Emergency Medicine

James Shen, Linda Ding, Kevin O'Connor, Ameer Elaimy, Carla Bradford, Fenhong Liu, Abdulnasser Khalifeh, Suhong Yu, Harry Bushe, Jonathan Saleeby, Kenneth Ulin, I-Lin Kuo, Yankhua Fan, Maryann Bishop-Jodoin, Paul Rava and Thomas J. FitzGerald

Abstract

The discovery of radiation has led to many advances. Guidelines have been created to minimize radiation exposure and treatment management following both unintentional and intentional exposure. The effects of radiation exposure on specific tissues varies. Tragic consequences can result, ranging from severe, acute injury to long- lasting effects that present years after the initial exposure. In this chapter we provide observations that demonstrate the importance of understanding guidelines to minimize radioactive exposure and the expectations and treatment management following exposure. For the safety and well-being of patients, health care professionals need to remain well-informed to minimize the risks of this tool.

Keywords: radiation injury, emergency care and treatment

1. Introduction

Our understanding of toxicity associated with exposure to radiation has increased since the discovery of X-rays in 1895. X-rays were used to treat a variety of malignant and non-malignant diseases. The effects of radioactive exposure on specific tissues can vary. Radioactive particles destroy or impair tissue by generating free radicals that damage important molecular structures, such as DNA. Radiation exposure can lead to catastrophic consequences, ranging from severe, acute injury to long-lasting effects that manifest years after the initial exposure. This chapter provides observations that demonstrate the importance of understanding guidelines to minimize radioactive exposure, and the expectations and treatment management following exposure [1–3].

Exposure to radioactive particles is divided into intentional or unintentional causes. Notable intentional causes include the atomic weapons activated on Hiroshima and Nagasaki in Japan during World War II. The immediate injuries and fatalities were from the heat and mechanical force generated by the trauma and physical destruction. However, it became apparent that there were longer lasting consequences. Survivors in the surrounding area were exposed to high levels of radiation and suffered from acute toxicity injuries and organ failure. Many of those who did not succumb to the effects of acute toxicity were known to suffer lifelong chronic conditions, such as developmental problems in newborns and increased cancer risk [4–6].

Unintentional causes are usually the result of radiation exposure without intent to injure. These unintentional causes are typically related to the effects of radioactive materials utilized for energy or medical treatment. The first radiograph was taken in 1895 and early pioneers in the field were unaware of the consequences of exposure. Initial procedures were often associated with unintentional exposure and were fraught with numerous complications such as skin blistering, hair loss and systemic toxicity that we now know were due to radiation toxicity. These signs and symptoms were similar to those present in exposed workers in the first nuclear development programs, many of whom would later develop injuries and cancers as a consequence of their profession [7, 8].

Despite these risks, nuclear power continues to be used for its benefits. Fortunately, we now know much more about how to avoid and minimize radioactive exposure. Rigorous standards enforcing safe practices with radioactive material and the formation of numerous regulatory agencies such as the Nuclear Regulatory Commission are a testament to how far we have come [9]. However, accidents involving radioactive material do occur. In this chapter, we describe a brief history of well-known incidents involving unintended radioactive exposure, as well as the clinical consequences and care of the patient following exposure.

2. Unintended causes: nuclear accidents

One of the most significant nuclear accidents in history was Chernobyl. On that day, a series of missteps during a routine safety check resulted in a massive explosion that sent a plume of radioactive material into the air for an entire week. The range of this explosion extended well beyond the immediate vicinity, exposing other parts of Europe to radioactive gas in the process. In addition to exposing civilians to the radioactive material, first responders also received significant radiation levels and thermal injury, many of which were lethal. More recently, the nuclear reactor in Fukushima, Japan experienced a meltdown following the 2011 tsunami in Japan. While there were no immediate casualties, there was lasting environmental damage and the long-term health consequences are yet to be fully understood [8]. These examples demonstrate the importance of proper safety measures and providing an effective response to nuclear accidents.

3. Acute toxicity

Toxicity from radiation exposure can be divided into three types: acute, subacute and chronic/late. Acute radiation toxicity is defined as signs and symptoms ≤90 days following exposure. In a medical setting, treatment of acute exposure is quite common. During radiation therapy, radiation is targeted and delivered to tumors and management of side effects from the radiation exposure remains a mainstay of modern oncology.

The radioactive dose from these procedures is typically far less than the dose following unintended exposures outside of the clinical setting. The radiation treatment dose is usually fractionated, meaning the dose is given in intervals to reduce the short-term toxicity of the radioactive treatment. The clinical manifestations of acute toxicity following a radioactive accident may be much more severe than those typically encountered by most physicians and may warrant treatment in an emergency setting [4, 5].

Acute radiation toxicity involves many organ systems, including but not limited to the central nervous, gastrointestinal, and cardiovascular systems. Cells with self-renewal potential may be able to recover better from radiation damage compared to those without such protective mechanisms. Self-renewal processes are often accelerated as a response to injury where slowly proliferative tissues cannot. However, if the exposure is given in a single fraction of high enough dose, this ability for self-renewal potential will be overwhelmed. For example, a single total body dose >10 Gy will result in death within days from numerous possible causes. Damage to the central nervous system will result in cerebrovascular syndrome, with uncontrollable swelling in neuromuscular tissue. Despite best supportive care there are no medical interventions to prevent death at this level of exposure. Damage to the gastrointestinal system results in severe diarrhea and associated fluid loss. The mechanism involves depletion of most stem cells within the gastrointestinal crypts. Since these stem cells are required to replace the mucosal surface, these mucosal surfaces will disappear a few days after exposure and there will be no barrier to prevent fluid loss or bacterial entrance into the bloodstream. As a result, patients will typically present with fever, nausea, vomiting, fatigue, anorexia, and severe hypotension. Doses of 4–5 Gy are enough to cause death from depleted stem cells in the hematopoietic system without support. Those that survive the initial depletion typically succumb to infection a month later due to depleted lymphocytes and other immune elements. These manifestations can occur minutes after exposure, with severity being proportional to dose and a sharp decrease in lymphocytes within two days of exposure [1, 4, 5].

Should the patient be exposed to doses below 4 Gy, symptomatic and best supportive treatment is recommended. Nausea and vomiting are the typical initial symptoms and should be treated with hydration. If the exposure dose is unknown, noting the time of onset of vomiting is important as exposure dose is inversely proportional to time to emesis. It is not uncommon for patients at low exposure doses to feel fine for a few weeks before the gastrointestinal and hematopoietic symptoms drive a patient to seek medical care. Upon initiation of care, isolation and contact inhibition is vital since infection is a major contributor towards death in these patients as depletion of the hematopoietic system occurs. Blood transfusion and antibiotics can be delivered to alleviate these issues. A patient will often also present with skin injury burns at the site of radiation exposure as epidermal and dermal injury associated with stem cell depletion can mimic and appear similar to a thermal injury. These injuries should be treated promptly, as they are easy routes for infection to occur, which can be devastating to a patient with a compromised hematopoietic system. In patients with high exposure doses, end of life care is a possible consideration. At an exposure of 5 Gy, only about half of patients will survive after 30 days. An exposure of 10 Gy is considered lethal regardless of medical interventions [1, 5, 6]. Treating patients following radiation exposure is not only challenging in terms of clinical aspects, but emotionally as well.

Compounds that have been developed to reduce and even prevent the clinical manifestations following radiation exposure are called mitigators. These compounds work by altering the molecular response following radiation exposure. As such, a mitigator could inhibit lymphocyte recruitment at sites of radiation damage, increase proliferation of stem cells that would normally be inhibited by radiation exposure, or inhibit fibrosis. An example of a mitigator is Palifermin, a growth factor that stimulates cell growth in response to radiation exposure to reduce recovery time. Radioprotectors, on the other hand, are given before or immediately after radiation exposure to protect against the effects of radiation toxicity [10, 11]. Amifostone is one such radioprotector that has been approved by the FDA for reducing side effects from radiation therapy [12]. More mitigators and radioprotectors are expected to be approved as the need to protect against radiation toxicity increases. Although many compounds have been and are in development, no others to date are actively used in clinical practice and the role of both hematopoietic and mesenchymal transplant remains under investigation.

4. Subacute and late toxicity

The subacute and/or late effects of radiation toxicity, by nature, are less visible and harder to identify for most emergency and primary care physicians. Often, these effects take many years to develop and are often mistaken as sequelae from another disease. However, they are nevertheless important to identify and address. A common misconception is that the degree to which a patient suffers from acute symptoms is proportional to severity of the long-term response. Unfortunately, patients who experience little to no acute sequela can experience serious long-term sequela, and vice versa. While both children and adults can experience the effects of late radiation toxicity, children are susceptible as they have a much longer period for these clinical manifestations to develop [13]. Unlike acute toxicity effects, anticipating long term effects is much more difficult. This technique relies heavily not only on a physician's knowledge of potential long-term effects, but also their willingness to investigate a potential long-term effect.

5. Organ specific injury

A common theme in radiation injury is the ability of the tissue or organ to respond to cell death and self-regenerate. These aspects vary among organs and thus the clinical presentation and treatment is different depending on the organ involved. Injuries and treatment protocols for specific organs are as follows:

5.1 Hematopoietic system

As previously discussed, damage to the hematopoietic system typically results from injury to progenitor cells, which can lead to hematopoietic crisis and infection. Fortunately, with the exception of whole-body exposure, the hematopoietic system is generally able to recover from radiation damage due to migration of stem cells from outside the site of exposure. Patients who are also receiving chemotherapy or taking medications that may result in immunosuppressed states should be carefully assessed. In the case of total body irradiation, an immediate decrease in circulating lymphocytes can be expected with subsequent defects in immune response. Symptomatic treatment, including blood infusions and antibiotics as needed, with isolation are crucial in these situations [13, 14]. Use of bone marrow transplants to replenish depleted progenitor cells has a theoretical survival benefit opportunity in total body irradiation patients, but to date has not been embraced as standard practice and often only applied to those most severely affected. The risk of graft-vs-host disease makes this approach controversial, especially in the setting of an emergency unrelated allogeneic transplant [6].

5.2 Skin

The skin is often the most direct site of radiation injury, as the epidermis covers all other organs and is susceptible to radiation damage. The dermal stem cells are the most susceptible component of the skin, as these are the actively dividing cells that replace other cells in the rest of the organ. Early symptoms of exposure typically involve erythema and swelling as vasodilation and the recruitment of inflammatory components localize to the area. These symptoms typically resolve within a month. Late term effects include decreased wound healing capacity with increased fibrosis and ulceration. Interestingly, the skin will appear to be more vascularized with more prominent vasculature. However, this is due to thinning of the epidermis, which causes veins to appear more prominent. Proper wound care is the standard treatment for these manifestations, with surgical debridement as needed. Particular concern must be paid for patients with medical conditions that are prone to fibrosis, such as those with dermatitis, lupus, and scleroderma. Skin infections, such as cellulitis, are particularly dangerous given the immunosuppressive effects of radiation therapy. Lastly, an interesting phenomenon occurs in some patients where previously irradiated skin can become erythemic and fibrotic several years later in response to certain medications like antibiotics and chemotherapy. The mechanism behind this phenomenon is unknown [15].

In the past, skin involvement from radiation therapy that could not be treated with topical ointments was relatively rare. However, with the increasing use of hypofractionation (radiation therapy with greater amounts of dose per treatment), these findings are becoming more common [16]. Thus, radiation damage to the skin is likely to become more prominent in the future as therapy becomes more compressed with higher doses delivered in a shorter period of time. Patients with a history of radiation therapy and significant skin sequalae should be carefully observed for more serious developments as injuries in treated tissues heal less well and contain less local immunity.

5.3 Gastrointestinal system

Like the skin, the gastrointestinal system is composed of mucosal cells with multiple layers underneath that are constantly replaced over time. Unfortunately, the rate at which some of these cells are replaced is higher than that of the skin, leading to more immediate and sometimes more severe clinical manifestations. Cells of the gastric and small bowel tend to have the highest rate of replacement, leading to very early nausea if these regions were exposed. Exposure to mucosal cells in the upper gastrointestinal system (mouth, esophagus, salivary glands) tend to present with clinical symptoms around two weeks after exposure due to a longer replacement rate. Damage to these cells tends to present with more localized pain and swelling. Exposure to the salivary glands can result not only with localized pain, but also xerostomia (dryness of mouth) and ageusia (loss of taste). Saliva can become more acidic which can further injure normal tissue and alter the environment of the oral cavity. Regardless of these manifestations, patients should be advised to maintain adequate nutrition and dental hygiene, as this practice helps mitigate the complications of an immunocompromised state. Symptomatic treatment of localized pain is also advised and considered standard of care as bone exposure can be a serious consequence of mucosal denudation [14]. **Figure 1** represents modern head/neck radiation therapy treatment plan through the oral cavity demonstrating sparing of the parotid tissue with intensity modulation.

Farther along the digestive tract, the expected symptoms can be predicted based on the location of the tumor. Radiation exposure to the gastric mucosa during treatment of gastric tumors can result in near immediate nausea given the daily replacement the gastric mucosa. Treatment of esophageal tumors, which are now more commonly in the lower third of the esophagus, present with a timeline of symptoms similar to head and neck tumors (approximately two weeks after exposure). Tumors in this region typically cause dysphagia and anorexia. Treatment initially tends to relieve patient symptoms, but later patients may return thinking the tumor

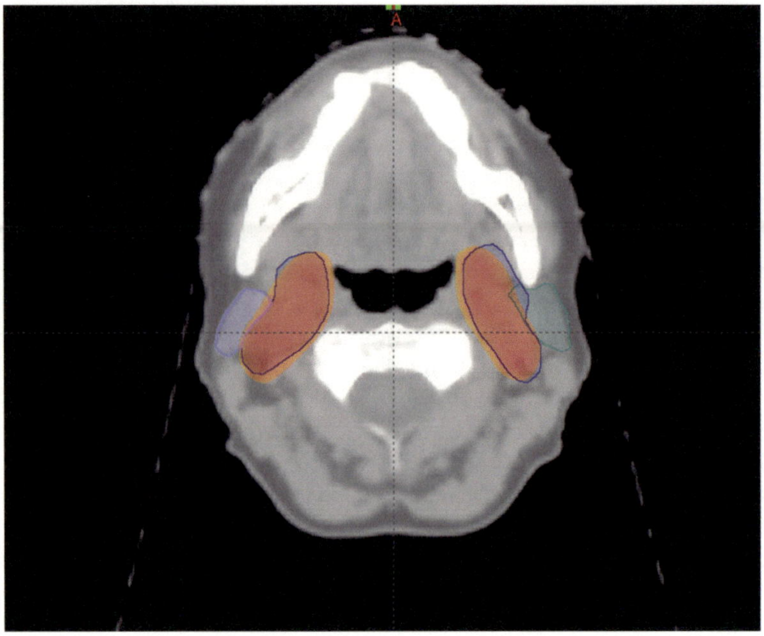

Figure 1.
Parotid sparing. Image courtesy of the Department of Radiation Oncology, University of Massachusetts Medical School.

has returned when in reality these symptoms are due to swelling from the therapy. Like head and neck tumors, patients should be advised to continue maintaining adequate hydration and nutrition [13, 14].

Symptoms from radiation exposure in the small and large bowel are more complex and require more in-depth patient history and laboratory tests. The small bowel absorbs much of the nutrients from food. Damaging the microvilli of the mucosal surface, which are vital for nutrient absorption, can result in severe malabsorption regardless of a patient's appetite. These findings can be confirmed by stool tests. Patients will often present to the emergency room with diarrhea, steatorrhea, bloating and general abdominal pain a few days after radiation exposure. The large bowel plays an important role in absorption of water, and exposure of large portions of this organ may compromise this function. Patients may complain of increased defecation frequency, which can lead to dehydration and electrolyte abnormalities that can be confirmed through electrolyte panels. To make matters more difficult, abdominal organs are prone to forming adhesions after surgical interventions, which disrupts blood flow to portions of the bowel that are exacerbated after concurrent radiation therapy. Anticipation of these issues through a careful patient history are vital to preventing severe complications from occurring [13, 14, 17].

Late effects of radiation also depend on location of the exposure. The mucosal cells of the oral cavity should theoretically recover like that of typical skin cells, but the combination of a tight space and harsh oral environment prone to infection and necrosis makes healing difficult. Thus, fibrosis and ulceration over a long period of time are possible. Acute effects of radiation typically damage mucosa of the gums and affect the pH of the saliva, facilitating microbial growth. These changes can lead to long-term problems with dental hygiene and patients should modify their dental habits accordingly through increased tooth brushing and fluoride mouthwash [13, 14]. Motility issues are also becoming more common, especially since patients who receive radiation therapy are now living longer. Dysphagia appears to be due to edema surrounding constrictor muscles, and physical therapy to encourage lymph drainage offers symptomatic treatment [18]. Gastric emptying issues due fibrosis at the gastric antrum and regions in the bowel where surgery was performed are also possible years after treatment. Atrophy of the pancreas many years after radiation exposure is also known to happen, although the clinical relevance of this is unknown [13, 14]. Symptoms can mimic malabsorption syndrome.

5.4 Lung

The main mechanism of radiation injury in the lungs is the generation of free oxygen and nitrogen radicals which damage the lung parenchyma with irregular repair of type I and II pneumocytes along the delicate reticulin network of pulmonary parenchyma. This oxidative damage causes disorganized repair and replacement of these cells associated with late fibrosis, impairs the ability for the lungs to oxygenate the blood. Pneumocyte damage also leads to recruitment of pro-inflammatory modulators that recruit immune cells to the region, leading to fibrosis and further depleting oxygenation capacity [19]. Furthermore, the radiation-driven production of nitric oxide has been suggested as a possible cause of damage to lung parenchyma outside of the field of radiation [20].

Complicating this situation is that many chemotherapeutic agents given with radiation therapy, such as bleomycin, also causes pulmonary fibrosis. The results of these sequelae are the development of pneumonitis up to two to six months after exposure. If asymptomatic, careful observation is standard of care. If symptomatic, the patient usually presents with occasional bouts of cough and dyspnea. Treatment with corticosteroids, supplementary oxygen, and prophylactic antibiotics are recommended in this situation. Once the pneumonitis resolves, fibrosis typically marks the site of radiation injury and can result in limited ventilation requiring long term use of supplemental oxygen. Given these findings, it is important to note that these patients tend to be at higher risk of developing chronic pulmonary disease compared to those who were unexposed [13, 21–24]. Pulmonary rehabilitation is an important aspect to survivorship care and optimizing respiratory health is important to each patient as the rehabilitate from therapy. **Figure 2** represents changes in lung parenchyma associated with immunotherapy and low dose radiation therapy with improvement seen after withdrawal of the immunotherapy.

5.5 Liver

Radiation injury to the liver, also known as radiation-induced liver disease (RILD), is unique in that it is often during the healing process that tissue function undergoes disorganized repair, including injury to the reticulum network, and limits the vascular relationship to the hepatocyte. While acute damage to hepatocytes affects liver function, as the cells divide during repair they tend to become disorganized, particularly if the structural reticulum of the liver is damaged. Increased distance between the hepatocytes and the blood supply leads to decreased liver function. This phenomenon explains why the state of the liver before exposure to radiation also plays an important role in this process. For example, a cirrhotic liver due to heavy alcoholic use or hepatitis will likely have pre-existing disorganized architecture, making this liver more susceptible to radiation damage. This includes veno-occlusive disease which also separates vascular anatomy from the hepatocyte. For these reasons, imaging studies such as magnetic resonance imaging before the delivery of radiation are obtained for evaluation of anatomy and function [25]. Disorganized repair can lead to migration of infusional therapies including radiolabeled therapy as the vascular anatomy can be disrupted and limit efficacy in spite of placement of therapy in close approximation to disease.

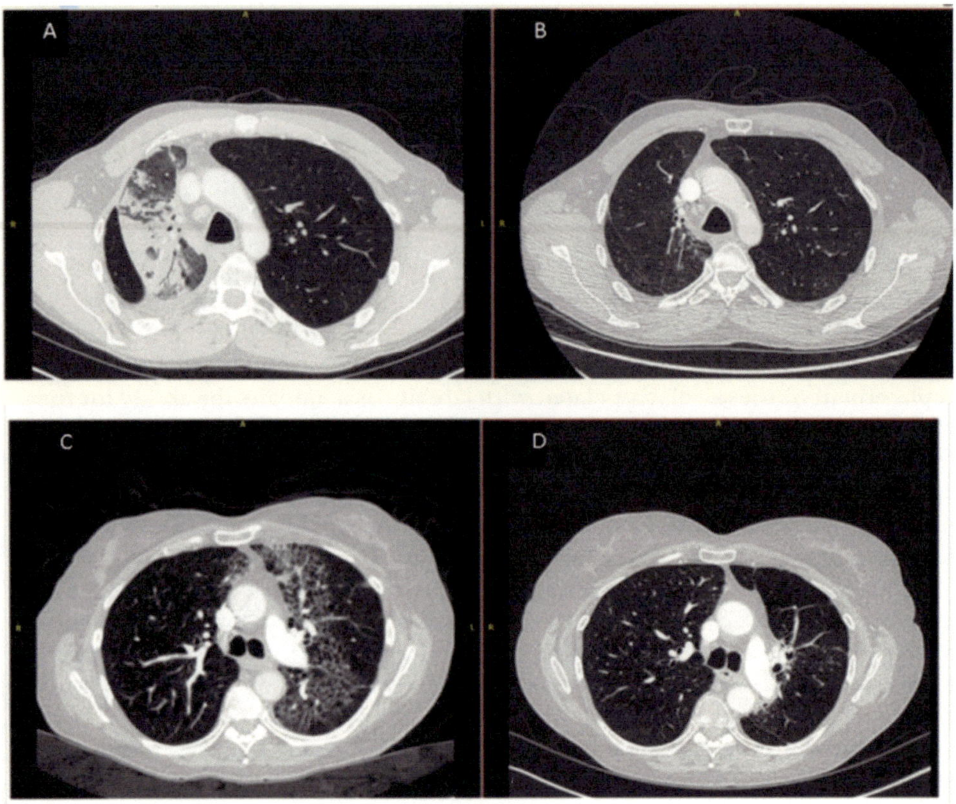

Figure 2.
(A) and (C) Therapy driven pneumonitis outlining the radiation therapy field while on immune check point inhibition. (B) and (D) Improvement after immunotherapy withdrawal. Courtesy of the Department of Radiation Oncology, University of Massachusetts Medical School.

Patients with RILD typically experience symptoms that mimic cirrhosis, which include abdominal pain, elevated liver enzymes, jaundice, and ascites within four months of radiation exposure. Livers with pre-existing damage typically have earlier onset, with more severe symptoms. Treatment is symptomatic with keen observation of potential veno-occlusive and metabolic disease secondary to a congested liver with decreased function. Careful consideration must be given for medications that are metabolized in the liver, especially chemotherapeutic agents that are also hepatotoxic [25, 26].

5.6 Renal

All components of the kidney, including structures crucial for filtration, such as cells of the glomerulus, are susceptible to radiation damage. The signs of acute radiation damage are usually seen within 3–18 months, typically mimicking signs of renal failure. These signs include decreased glomerular filtration rate (GFR), increased serum β2-microglobulin, albuminuria, and other markers of poor renal function. Later signs of kidney radiation damage, which include hypertension and eventual renal failure, are often hard to distinguish from other pathological causes. For treatment of these sequelae, the use of hypertension medications such as angiotensin-converting-enzyme inhibitors (ACE) inhibitors are theoretically beneficial. Monitoring of renal function, both short and long term, also remains crucial in the standard of care for these patients [27–29]. In aging patients who are

DOI: http://dx.doi.org/10.5772/intechopen.95262

not candidates for surgery, radiation therapy with stereotactic techniques is being used more frequently to treat sub-total renal volumes for renal malignancies in an effort to spare as much renal function as possible.

5.7 Cardiovascular system

The mechanism of radiation damage to the heart and blood vessels involves immediate cellular damage followed by fibrotic and disorganized repair, leading to reduced function in all cardiac segments including electrical conduction, myocardium, valves, and vascular anatomy. The time period is variable due to differences in size and functional architecture. However, what is clear is that unintended radiation exposure to the heart and blood vessels has a strong association with cardiovascular disease and complications [30–33]. The lack of mitigation and therapeutic strategies in response to radiation of cardiovascular tissues explains why radiation oncologists spend such a large amount of effort to minimize cardiovascular exposure [34].

Generous radiation exposure to the heart can result in acute pericarditis. This diagnosis should always be in the differential in a patient with history of radiation exposure who presents with sharp, radiating chest pain that is relieved when sitting up. Anti-inflammatory medications like aspirin, colchicine and prednisone can offer symptomatic relief, with pericardiocentesis being an option in severe cases. Long term, patients who receive radiation exposure to the heart have a higher risk of heart disease and use of echocardiograms and nuclear stress tests in these patients is recommended if symptoms warrant use. Large blood vessels like the aortic, carotid, and femoral arteries can experience hyperplasia and atherosclerotic change from radiation doses. These changes can result in rupture and fistula formation, necessitating immediate treatment. This usually requires very high doses and prolonged exposure usually not seen in modern radiation therapy [30–33]. With improvements in survival, patients can receive therapy with intentional overlap to previously treated volumes for second malignancies. These patients are vulnerable to vascular injury, including larger arteries and survivorship plans need to include periodic surveillance of vessels to optimize follow up care. **Figure 3** demonstrates cardiac sparing for left-sided breast cancer treatment with breath-hold treatment techniques and optical tracking.

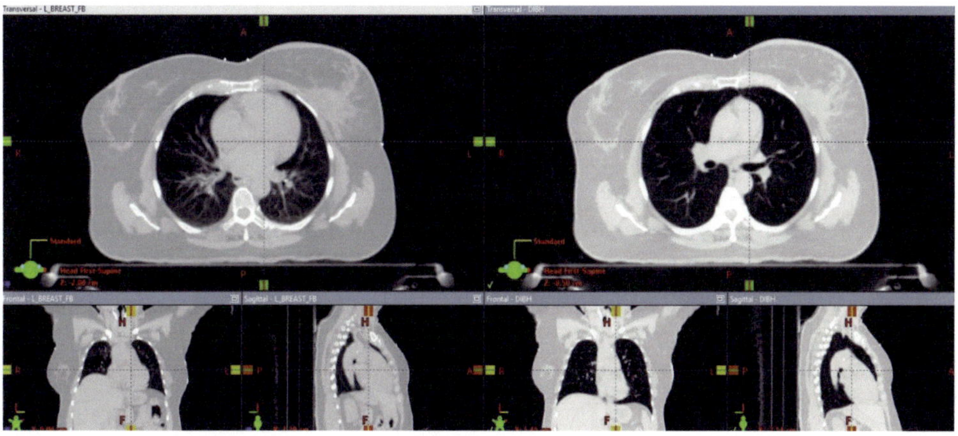

Figure 3.
Cardiac sparing with deep inspiration breath-hold (DIBH), (left-free-breathing (FB); right-DIBH). Image courtesy of the Department of Radiation Oncology, University of Massachusetts Medical School.

5.8 Nervous system

Since most cells of the nervous system do not typically have a high turnover rate, it would seem reasonable to assume that the nervous system is more resistant to radiation damage than other organs. However, this assumption does not account for the immediate molecular effects of radiation. Regardless of the rate of cell division, all cells will receive damage to membranes, organelles, and other structures within the cell. Cells that do not divide very frequently will have to endure these injuries for long periods of time, leading to eventual clinical manifestations. Damage to nearby vasculature also limits growth and healing of these structures, leading to pronounced long term effects. There are clear reports of radiation damage to the central nervous system sometimes long after the initial radiation exposure [35–38].

Patients who received radiosurgery or hypofractionation techniques are at risk of developing necrosis within six months of receiving therapy. Clinically, these developments can result in focal changes and change in behavior depending on the site of necrosis. Demyelinating syndromes, although rare, are also possible in the peripheral nerves and spinal cord. Often, neurotoxic symptoms are enhanced by chemotherapeutic agents, such as vinblastine, vincristine and cisplatin. Gathering a detailed physical exam, medical history and possible neurological referral may be required for definitive identification of these outcomes. Patients who received radiation therapy for pituitary adenomas or at sites near the optic structures are at risk for visual changes [36, 37]. This is because some structures, such as the lens and optic chasm, are sensitive to radiation exposure due to limited blood supply [15, 39, 40]. Patients treated for breast and head and neck cancers may rarely present with brachial plexopathy. Peripheral lymph nodes for these regions are often within the same field of treatment as the brachial plexus, resulting in unintended exposure to this region [41].

5.9 Endocrine

The effect of radiation therapy on the endocrine glands varies depending on the gland affected. The timeline for the development of clinical sequelae varies, with some cases even being reported many years after the radiation exposure. The pituitary gland is relatively radiation sensitive and results in panhypopituitary syndrome, requiring supplementation of depleted hormones. Secondary malignancies from un-intentional radiation exposure, while rare, have been reported [42]. Patients who received previous head and neck radiation therapy who now present with headache, vision loss and/or hormonal abnormalities should be carefully examined for the development of pituitary adenomas. The thyroid gland is also sensitive to radiation therapy, resulting in hypothyroid syndromes. Patients who receive radiation therapy to the head and neck often receive surgery that involves dissection of the thyroid gland, exasperating thyroid function loss. The thyroid also has a relatively higher incidence of developing secondary malignancies. This finding has been identified not only in patients receiving radiation therapy, but also victims of the Chernobyl incident [5]. The same care must be given to the parathyroid glands, given the proximity to the thyroid gland, which can present with signs and symptoms of hypoparathyroidism. Radiation exposure to the endocrine pancreas and adrenal glands are less characterized and are thought to be more radiation resistant. However, there are a few cases of injury to these organs associated with radiation exposure [42].

5.10 Reproductive

The reproductive organs are highly sensitive to radiation damage, with early exposure in pediatric patients leading to severe detriments like sterility and secondary malignancies (see Pediatrics). Since much of the reproductive system depends on hormonal homeostasis, radioactive effects on the endocrine system (see Endocrine) and the subsequent effect on hormone production, such as that on testosterone and estrogen, can drastically affect reproductive function and development depending on the effected hormone and gland. When investigating radiation injury to the reproductive system, it is always important to consider the location of exposure and any endocrine glands involved. Germ cells, such as spermatogonia, are particularly sensitive to radiation damage as they can experience inter-mitotic death. Even mild radiation exposure can lead to a heavy drop in sperm numbers. Mature sperm that receive radiation damage can harbor serious mutations or chromosomal abnormalities, leading to severe birth defects in progeny. Exposure to female reproductive organs can even lead to miscarriage and early menopause. As a result, it usually recommended for patients who receive gonadal exposure practice birth control methods for up to six months after the exposure. Because the ovaries rely on a regular, cyclical production of hormones from the follicles, radiation injury can lead to more pronounced effects on fertility. Mucosal atrophy and drying of female genitalia can cause great discomfort for the patient as well. Thus, fertility treatment and consultation should be considered for patients who received heavy or repeated radiation exposure to the gonads [13, 14, 42].

6. Pediatrics

Pediatric patients are unique in that many organs and tissues are still developing. As a result, the cells involved are particularly sensitive to radiation damage as the fully developed adult organ can become abnormal or dysfunctional. Pediatric patients who receive radiation therapy are known to have a higher risk of developing growth abnormalities, chronic diseases, secondary malignancies and premature death compared to sibling controls [43]. Children who were treated with radiotherapy in the pelvis for tumors such as rhabdomyosarcoma or germ cell tumors are at high risk for gonadal abnormalities. Given the rapid growth in the musculoskeletal system during puberty, exposure to the spine at an early age can cause drastic changes to the respiratory and cardiovascular system. Radiation exposure to any cartilage or bone not only presents the risk of bone necrosis, but also may affect the fully developed form of such tissue, sometimes resulting in stunted extremity length and increased frequency of fractures. Children treated for Wilms tumors are at high risk of renal abnormalities later in their lifetime to the remaining kidney, therefore attention to detail for renal health as these patients become adults is an important aspect of a survivorship plan. Exposure to the bowel and hepatic structures are known to adversely affect the growth and development of intraabdominal organs. These effects can affect nutritional intake, indirectly causing developmental issues as the child matures [14, 43, 44]. As these patients mature into adulthood, detailed review of a patient's radiation exposure history will play a pivotal role in survivorship plans.

7. Mitigation strategies in planning

As many of the side effects of radiation therapy are difficult to anticipate and manage, a great deal of effort has been put into reducing the amount of non-tumor tissue exposed to radiation. In the early days of radiation, this was difficult simply due to the lack of technology. Now, most radiation oncologists have access to various new tools, such as 4-dimensional conformal avoidance techniques to minimize off-target exposure [34]. Compact structures that were traditionally difficult to irradiate without significant off-target, such as the axilla and chest, can now be treated much more accurately with minimal exposure to non-tumor tissue [41]. Modern imaging techniques can be utilized to assess organ performance even before the administration of radiation to determine the risk of post-radiation symptoms. Indocyanine retention assays used in conjunction with MRI have determined the pre-exposure function of liver to assess if the patient is a good candidate for radiation therapy [25]. New guidelines are constantly being updated to ensure that the risks of radiation therapy are minimized. Novel pharmacological agents, such as the development of immunotherapy, are being implemented to supplement the efficiency of radiation therapy. As medicine becomes more collaborative and data is more available, physicians outside of radiation oncology will be able to better understand the radiation therapy treatment plans and define survivorship care plans accordingly.

8. Conclusions

The discovery of nuclear power and the utilization to benefit humanity has been one of the defining moments of the modern era. While this discovery certainly has benefits, there are also unintended and intended consequences which we must continue to mitigate. In the field of medicine, what is clear is that radiation remains a crucial tool to diagnose and treat diseases. Understanding and minimizing the risks of using this tool remains a priority for the safety and well-being of patients, especially given the broad impact it has on organs throughout the body and the long-term effects. It falls upon health care professionals to remain vigilant and well-informed to ensure that nuclear energy and radiation therapy remains a blessing and not a curse.

Conflict of interest

The authors declare no conflict of interest.

Author details

James Shen[1], Linda Ding[2], Kevin O'Connor[1], Ameer Elaimy[1], Carla Bradford[2], Fenhong Liu[2], Abdulnasser Khalifeh[3], Suhong Yu[3], Harry Bushe[2], Jonathan Saleeby[2], Kenneth Ulin[1], I-Lin Kuo[2], Yankhua Fan[2], Maryann Bishop-Jodoin[1], Paul Rava[2] and Thomas J. FitzGerald[2*]

1 University of Massachusetts Medical School, Worcester, MA, USA

2 University of Massachusetts Medical School, UMass Memorial Health Care, Worcester, MA, USA

3 UMass Memorial Health Care, Worcester, MA, USA

*Address all correspondence to: tj.fitzgerald@umassmemorial.org

References

[1] Hall EJ, Giaccia AJ, editors. Radiobiology for the Radiologist. 7th ed. Philadelphia: Lippincott, Williams and Wilkins; 2012.

[2] Miller DL, Balter S, Cole PE, Lu HT, Berenstein A, Albert R, et al. Radiation doses in interventional radiology procedures: the RAD-IR study: part II: Skin dose. J Vasc Interv Radiol. 2003;14(8):977-990.

[3] Miller DL, Balter S, Wagner LK, Cardella J, Clark TW, Neithamer CD, Jr., et al. Quality improvement guidelines for recording patient radiation dose in the medical record. J Vasc Interv Radiol. 2004;15(5):423-429.

[4] Donnelly EH, Nemhauser JB, Smith JM, Kazzi ZN, Farfan EB, Chang AS, et al. Acute radiation syndrome: assessment and management. South Med J. 2010;103(6):541-546.

[5] Turai I, Veress K. Radiation accidents: occurrence, types, consequences, medical management, and lessons learned. Central Eur J Occup Environ Med. 2001;7(1):3-14.

[6] Baranov A, Gale RP, Guskova A, Piatkin E, Selidovkin G, Muravyova L, et al. Bone marrow transplantation after the Chernobyl nuclear accident. N Engl J Med. 1989;321(4):205-212.

[7] Sansare K, Khanna V, Karjodkar F. Early victims of X-rays: A tribute and current perception. Dentomaxillofacial Radiology. 2011;40:123-125. DOI: 101259dmfr/73488299.

[8] Lushbagh CC, Ricks RC, Fry SA. Radiological accidents: A historical review of sealed source accidents. In: Proceedings of the International Conference on Radiation Protection in Nuclear Energy. Sydney (Australia): US Nuclear Regulatory Commission; April 18-22, 1988; IAEA-CN-51/92. 1988; 522.

[9] International Atomic Energy Agency. Scientific and Technical Basis for the Geological Disposal of Radioactive Wastes. Technical Reports Series 413. 2003. STI/DOC/010/413. ISBN: 92-0-100103-7.

[10] Citrin D, Cotrim AP, Hyodo F, Baum BJ, Krishna MC, Mitchell JB. Radioprotectors and mitigators of radiation-induced normal tissue injury. Oncologist. 2010;15(4):360-371.

[11] Radtke ML, Kolesar JM. Palifermin (Kepivance) for the treatment of oral mucositis in patients with hematologic malignancies requiring hematopoietic stem cell support. J Oncol Pharm Pract. 2005;11(3):121-125. doi:10.1191/1078155205jp159oa.

[12] Brizel DM, Wasserman TH, Henke M, Strnad V, Rudat V, Monnier A, et al. Phase III randomized trial of amifostine as a radioprotector in head and neck cancer. J Clin Oncol. 2000;18(19):3339-3345.

[13] Bentzen SM. Preventing or reducing late side effects of radiation therapy: radiobiology meets molecular pathology. Nat Rev Cancer. 2006;6(9):702-713.

[14] FitzGerald TJ, Aronowitz J, Giulia Cicchetti M, Fisher G, Kadish S, Lo YC, et al. The effect of radiation therapy on normal tissue function. Hematol Oncol Clin North Am. 2006;20(1):141-163.

[15] Fitzgerald TJ, Jodoin MB, Tillman G, Aronowitz J, Pieters R, Balducci S, et al. Radiation therapy toxicity to the skin. Dermatol Clin. 2008;26(1):161-172, ix.

[16] Hoppe BS, Laser B, Kowalski AV, Fontenla SC, Pena-Greenberg E, Yorke ED, et al. Acute skin toxicity following stereotactic body radiation therapy for stage I non-small-cell lung cancer: who's at risk? Int J Radiat Oncol Biol Phys. 2008;72(5):1283-1286.

[17] Moulder JE, Cohen EP. Future strategies for mitigation and treatment of chronic radiation-induced normal tissue injury. Semin Radiat Oncol. 2007;17(2):141-148.

[18] McCulloch TM, Jaffe D. Head and neck disorders affecting swallowing. GI Motility. 2006. DOI: doi:10.1038/gimo36.

[19] Rosiello RA, Merrill WW. Radiation-induced lung injury. Clin Chest Med. 1990;11(1):65-71.

[20] Sugihara T, Hattori Y, Yamamoto Y, Qi F, Ichikawa R, Sato A, et al. Preferential impairment of nitric oxide-mediated endothelium-dependent relaxation in human cervical arteries after irradiation. Circulation. 1999;100(6):635-641.

[21] Armstrong GT, Kawashima T, Leisenring W, Stratton K, Stovall M, Hudson MM, et al. Aging and risk of severe, disabling, life-threatening, and fatal events in the childhood cancer survivor study. J Clin Oncol. 2014;32(12):1218-1227.

[22] Hanania AN, Mainwaring W, Ghebre YT, Hanania NA, Ludwig M. Radiation-Induced Lung Injury: Assessment and Management. Chest. 2019;156(1):150-162.

[23] Rajan Radha R, Chandrasekharan G. Pulmonary injury associated with radiation therapy - Assessment, complications and therapeutic targets. Biomed Pharmacother. 2017;89:1092-1104.

[24] Giuranno L, Ient J, De Ruysscher D, Vooijs MA. Radiation-Induced Lung Injury (RILI). Front Oncol. 2019;9:877. DOI: 10.3389/fonc.2019.00877.

[25] Guha C, Kavanagh BD. Hepatic radiation toxicity: avoidance and amelioration. Semin Radiat Oncol. 2011;21(4):256-263.

[26] Pan CC, Kavanagh BD, Dawson LA, Li XA, Das SK, Miften M, et al. Radiation-associated liver injury. Int J Radiat Oncol Biol Phys. 2010;76(3 Suppl):S94-100.

[27] Dawson LA, Kavanagh BD, Paulino AC, Das SK, Miften M, Li XA, et al. Radiation-associated kidney injury. Int J Radiat Oncol Biol Phys. 2010;76(3 Suppl):S108-115.

[28] Cohen EP, Robbins ME. Radiation nephropathy. Semin Nephrol. 2003;23(5):486-499.

[29] Bolling T, Ernst I, Pape H, Martini C, Rube C, Timmermann B, et al. Dose-volume analysis of radiation nephropathy in children: preliminary report of the risk consortium. Int J Radiat Oncol Biol Phys. 2011;80(3):840-844.

[30] Evans SB, Sioshansi S, Moran MS, Hiatt J, Price LL, Wazer DE. Prevalence of poor cardiac anatomy in carcinoma of the breast treated with whole-breast radiotherapy: reconciling modern cardiac dosimetry with cardiac mortality data. Am J Clin Oncol. 2012;35(6):587-592.

[31] Lenihan DJ, Cardinale DM. Late cardiac effects of cancer treatment. J Clin Oncol. 2012;30(30):3657-3664.

[32] Marks LB, Yu X, Prosnitz RG, Zhou SM, Hardenbergh PH, Blazing M, et al. The incidence and functional consequences of RT-associated cardiac perfusion defects. Int J Radiat Oncol Biol Phys. 2005;63(1):214-223.

[33] Yusuf SW, Sami S, Daher IN. Radiation-induced heart disease: a clinical update. Cardiol Res Pract. 2011;2011:317659. DOI: 10.4061/2011/317659.

[34] Moslehi J. The cardiovascular perils of cancer survivorship. N Engl J Med. 2013;368(11):1055-1056.

[35] Pieters RS, Niemierko A, Fullerton BC, Munzenrider JE. Cauda equina tolerance to high-dose fractionated irradiation. Int J Radiat Oncol Biol Phys. 2006;64(1):251-257.

[36] Giese W, Kinsella T. Radiation injury to peripheral and cranial nerves. In: Gutin P, Leibel S, G S, editors. Radiation Injury to the Nervous System. New York: Raven; 1991. p. 383-403.

[37] Greene-Schloesser D, Moore E, Robbins ME. Molecular pathways: radiation-induced cognitive impairment. Clin Cancer Res. 2013;19(9):2294-2300.

[38] Ahles TA, Root JC, Ryan EL. Cancer- and cancer treatment-associated cognitive change: an update on the state of the science. J Clin Oncol. 2012;30(30):3675-3686.

[39] Harris JR, Levene MB. Visual complications following irradiation for pituitary adenomas and craniopharyngiomas. Radiology. 1976;120(1):167-171.

[40] Stoll BA, Andrews JT. Radiation-induced Peripheral neuropathy. Br Med J. 1966;1(5491):834-837.

[41] Powell S, Cooke J, Parsons C. Radiation-induced brachial plexus injury: follow-up of two different fractionation schedules. Radiother Oncol. 1990;18(3):213-220.

[42] Niazi AK, Niazi SK. Endocrine effects of Fukushima: Radiation-induced endocrinopathy. Indian J Endocrinol Metab. 2011;15(2):91-95.

[43] Armstrong GT, Kawashima T, Leisenring W, Stratton K, Stovall M, Hudson MM, et al. Aging and risk of severe, disabling, life-threatening, and fatal events in the childhood cancer survivor study. J Clin Oncol. 2014;32(12):1218-1227.

[44] Hopewell JW. Radiation-therapy effects on bone density. Med Pediatr Oncol. 2003;41(3):208-211.

Chapter 2

Evaluation and Treatment of Elevated Temperature in the Emergency Department

Marina Boushra

Abstract

Elevated patient temperature is a common vital sign abnormality in the emergency department that can be caused either by fever or hyperthermia. Fever is a frequent presentation, most commonly caused by infections of the respiratory or urinary tracts. Other occult sources include musculoskeletal, cardiac, neurological, and intra-abdominal infections. These infections can become complicated by sepsis and septic shock, conditions with high mortality. Treatment of the febrile acutely-ill patient should begin with fluids, antimicrobials, and source control. However, if this is ineffective or if the presentation is inconsistent with infection, consideration should be given to hyperthermia, rather than fever, being the cause of the patient's elevated temperature. Several life-threatening and reversible conditions can mimic sepsis and present with elevated temperature. These mimics include toxicity from medications and illicit substances, neuroleptic malignant syndrome, malignant hyperthermia, and thyroid storm. Identification of these mimics as the source of elevated temperature can lead to earlier diagnosis and improved outcomes in these patients.

Keywords: fever, hyperthermia, sepsis, overdose, infection

1. Introduction: fever vs. hyperthermia

Elevated core body temperature is a common vital sign abnormality in the emergency department (ED) that can be caused by fever or hyperthermia. While both *fever* and *hyperthermia* describe a state of elevated core temperature, they are pathophysiologically distinct clinical entities with different underlying pathologies and treatments. Fever is defined as an elevated body temperature that occurs secondary to a normal thermoregulatory system functioning at a higher set point in response to a stimulus, most commonly infection or inflammation [1]. In contrast, hyperthermia causes elevated body temperature through primary dysfunction of the hypothalamic thermoregulatory system itself [1]. Fever accounts for the vast majority of cases of elevated core temperature presentations in the ED, while hyperthermia is much more rare [1, 2]. Distinguishing between fever and hyperthermia may be difficult on initial patient presentation to the ED but the distinction has important implications for patient treatment and outcomes.

2. Fever

Fever results from a pyrogen-mediated alteration in the set point of the thermoregulatory system in the anterior hypothalamus [1]. The interaction of endogenous and exogenous pyrogens with the hypothalamus results in increased production of prostaglandins, which act on temperature-sensitive neurons and lead to increased core temperature [1] Infection is the most common cause of fever, accounting for 74% of fevers in hospitalized patients [3]. Other processes that produce endogenous pyrogens, such as malignancy and ischemia, account for the majority of the remaining sources of fever in hospitalized medical patients [4].

2.1 Sepsis

2.1.1 Definition of sepsis and septic shock

Despite significant emphasis by the Centers of Medicare and Medicaid Services (CMS) on the rapid identification and treatment of sepsis, there is no gold standard definition for the spectrum of sepsis syndromes. In actuality, sepsis is a complex and poorly understood process despite two centuries of research into its mechanisms. Sepsis is thought to result from a dysregulated and overexaggerated immune response to infection [5]. However, the complexity of sepsis and the variability in its presentation has thus far defied the creation of a gold standard definition, despite nearly three decades of attempts. The first definition of sepsis spectrum disorders was published in 1992 as a joint consensus statement between the American College of Chest Physicians (ACCP) and the Society of Critical Care Medicine (SCCM) [6]. This first consensus definition defined the presence sepsis spectrum disorders on elements of the patient's systemic inflammatory response syndrome (SIRS) (**Table 1**) [6]. This definition had poor sensitivity and specificity for sepsis spectrum disorders, and multiple guidelines have since attempted to revise these initial definitions, with variable success in increasing the sensitivity and specificity. The most recent consensus definition, Sepsis-3, was published in 2016 by SSCM and the European Society of Intensive Care Medicine (ESCIM) and defined the sepsis spectrum disorders by the presence of infection and two or more elements of the quick Sequential Organ Failure Assessment (qSOFA) [7]. The Sepsis-3 consensus definitions are outlined in **Table 2** below [7].

SIRS	Two or more of the following: Temperature > 38°C or < 36°C Heart rate > 90 beats per minute Respiratory rate > 20 breaths per minute or PaCO2 < 32 mmHg White blood cell count >12,000 cu/mm, <4000 cu/mm, >10% bands
Sepsis	Two SIRS criteria in the setting of known or suspected infection.
Severe sepsis	Sepsis and end-organ dysfunction
Septic shock	Sepsis with a systolic blood pressure < 90 mmHg or > 40 mmHg decrease in baseline systolic blood pressure

Table 1.
Defining sepsis based on systemic inflammatory response syndrome (SIRS): Adapted from the 1992 ACCP/SCCM consensus statement [6].

qSOFA	Altered mental status Systolic blood pressure < 90 mmHg Respiratory rate ≥ 22 breaths per minute

Table 2.
Quick sequential organ failure assessment criteria (qSOFA) [7]: sepsis-3 defines sepsis as infection with two or more of the components listed below.

2.1.2 Guidelines for the management of sepsis spectrum disorders

The Surviving Sepsis Campaign (SSC) guidelines offer recommendations for the resuscitation of patients with suspected sepsis spectrum disorders [8]. However, while these guidelines can provide an overview for the care of these patients, treatment should always be primarily guided by repeated clinical assessment and reassessment of these patients. Current guidelines recommend the continuous administration of crystalloid fluids as long as hemodynamic factors continue to improve [8] If 30 ml/kg ideal body weight (IBW) balanced crystalloid fluids does not achieve a MAP ≥65 mm Hg, a vasoactive agent should be started [8]. Norepinephrine is currently the vasopressor of choice patients with septic shock [8]. The cornerstone of management of sepsis spectrum disorders is prompt source control through administration of antimicrobials or, if necessary, surgical intervention [8]. Cultures should be collected before the first dose of antimicrobial medications; culture collection should not delay source control interventions [8]. In the emergency department, early broad-spectrum antimicrobial therapy should be initiated based on the pathogen profile of the suspected site of infection, the patient's prior culture results and susceptibilities, and local pathogen prevalence and resistance patterns. The spectrum of the antimicrobial agents can be narrowed as culture results become available or the patient presentation changes. Input from clinical pharmacists in the ED can assist in optimizing the initial antimicrobial choice and has been shown to decrease time to antibiotic administration, improve antibiotic stewardship, and improve patient outcomes [9–12].

2.2 Common sources: respiratory and urinary tract

Infections of the lower respiratory and urinary tracts comprise the majority of sepsis presentations to the ED. Community-acquired pneumonia (CAP) can be caused by a variety of bacterial and viral pathogens, with *Strepotococcus pneumoniae* being the most common bacterial etiology in those requiring hospitalization [13]. Other commonly implicated organisms include *Haemophilus influenzae, Mycoplasma pneumoniae,* and respiratory viruses. In patients requiring admission to a critical care unit, *S. pneumoniae* is still the most common etiologic organism but *Legionella pneumophila, Staphylococcus aureus,* gram-negative bacilli and influenza virus are more common [14]. Risk factors for drug resistance in CAP include age > 65, alcoholism, medical comorbidities, immunocompromise, immunosuppressive medication use, and use of beta-lactam, macrolide, or fluorquinolone antibiotics in the last 3–6 months [15]. Patients with hospitalization within three months have increased risk for hospital-acquired pneumonia with nosocomial organisms and their antibiotic regimens should include adequate coverage for *Staphylococcus aureus* and *Psuedomonas auerginosa,* which are more common in this population [15].

Infections of the urinary tract account for 40% of cases of nosocomial sepsis and the risk of infection is greatest in patients with structural or functional genitourinary abnormalities [16]. Sepsis from urinary source is more common in females [17].

Uncomplicated cystitis and pyelonephritis in women is typically caused by *Escherichia coli,* though *Proteus mirabilis, Klebsiella pneumoniae,* and *Streptococcus saprophyticus* are also relatively common [18]. As such, empiric treatment for uncomplicated urinary tract infections is best tailored to the regional *E. coli* sensitivities [18]. A complicated urinary tract infection is one which is associated with a condition that increases the risk for therapeutic failure [19]. These risk factors include diabetes, pregnancy, ureterolithiasis, renal failure, >7 days of symptoms, or an indwelling urinary device [19]. The microbial spectrum of complicated UTI is more varied and includes not only the typical organisms associated with uncomplicated UTI but also *Pseudomonas, Staphylococcus*, and *Serratia* species as well as fungi [19]. Complicated lower urinary tract infections may be managed as an outpatient; indications for hospitalization include inability to tolerate oral therapy or suspected infection with an organism resistant to oral therapies, such as extended-spectrum beta-lactamase producing organisms (ESBLs) [19].

2.3 Musculoskeletal

A comprehensive physical examination is of utmost importance in patients with a potential musculoskeletal infection as laboratory evaluation in these patients is generally non-diagnostic. Poor circulation and neuropathy are important risk factors for the development of musculoskeletal infections, and, as such, patients may not be able localize the source of their infection. Examination should include turning the patient to examine the back, palpation of the large joints, and examination of the feet and genitourinary regions for skin changes, which are often the only clue to the presence of a musculoskeletal infection [20, 21]. Comparison with the contralateral side can help to provide a baseline with which to compare for abnormalities. Practitioners should also evaluate for the presence of decubitus ulcers, which can become a nidus for osteomyelitis or bacteremia. Crepitus or pain out of proportion to examination should prompt concern for necrotizing soft tissue infection. Erythema, swelling, or pain with passive motion in a joint are concerning for a septic joint, with the knee and hip being the most common sources [22]. Risk factors for musculoskeletal infections include vasculopathy, diabetes, surgery, and immunocompromise [20]. *Staphylococcus aureus* or *Streptococcus pyogenes*-associated cellulitis is the most common cause of sepsis secondary to musculoskeletal infection [20]. While magnetic resonance imaging (MRI), surgical pathology, or culture is often necessary for the definitive diagnosis of most musculoskeletal infections, this should not delay early and aggressive source control in the ED.

2.4 Cardiac

Infectious pericarditis, myocarditis, and endocarditis as causes of sepsis can be easily missed in the emergency department due to their often subtle and variable presentations. Acute infectious pericarditis describes infection of the fibrous tissue encasing the heart and the base of the aorta and vena cava. Echoviruses and coxsackie A and B viruses account for nearly 90% of cases of infective pericarditis, with bacterial, parasitic, and fungal organisms accounting for the minority of cases [23]. The most common bacterial pathogens implicated in infective pericarditis are *Streptococcus pneumoniae* and *Staphylococcus auresus* [23]. The diagnosis of acute pericarditis is based on the presence of characteristic chest pain and electrocardiographic abnormalities [23]. Auscultation of a friction rub is helpful but is poorly sensitive for the diagnosis [24]. Infective myocarditis describes infection of the myocardial tissue, with coxsackie B being the most common cause. Other common causes include influenza virus, adenovirus, hepatitis C virus, parvovirus

B-19, and cytomegalovirus [23]. Infectious myocarditis should be considered in patients presenting with chest pain and signs of heart failure, especially when there is concurrent fever. Finally, the presence of a new murmur in an acutely ill patient should raise suspicion for infective endocarditis (IE), infection of endocardial lining of the heart valves. Important risk factors for endocarditis include intravenous drug use, prosthetic valves, indwelling intravascular devices, and immunocompromise [25]. IE presents remarkably variably and symptoms depend on the stage of disease. Fever is the most common symptom of IE; other findings concerning for endocarditis include stigmata of peripheral thromboembolism such as Osler nodes, Janeway lesions, Roth spots, or splinter hemorrhages [25]. Patients with IE may also present initially with complications of endocarditis, which include cerebrovascular ischemia or hemorrhage, septic emboli, and metastatic infection.

2.5 Meningitis and encephalitis

Meningitis is an infection of the meningeal lining of the central nervous system by bacteria, viruses, or fungi, with bacterial causes accounting the highest global burden [26]. Encephalitis describes infection of the cerebral parenchyma with a pathogen. *Streptococcus pneumonia,* group B streptococci, and *Neisseria meningitidis* are the most common causes of bacterial meningitis, with *Listeria monocytogenes* also being common in children, immunocompromised individuals, and adults greater than 50 years of age [26, 27]. Common viral causes of meningitis and encephalitis include herpesviruses, enteroviruses, and cytomegalovirus [28]. Fever, altered mental status, and nuchal rigidity are the classically described triad of meningitis, but the majority of patients in clinical practice only manifest one or two of these symptoms [26]. Lumbar puncture with cerebrospinal fluid (CSF) analysis is the diagnostic test of choice for meningitis. CT imaging should precede lumbar puncture in patients whose symptoms may be secondary to mass effect, such as those with immunocompromise, new seizure, papilledema, focal neurologic deficit, or altered mental status [26, 28, 29] Importantly, diagnostic studies should not delay the administration of antimicrobials in patients with suspected meningitis or encephalitis. Administration of antimicrobials prior to lumbar puncture has been shown to have minimal effect on chemistry and cytology findings studies of CSF but may lead to a falsely negative Gram stain or culture [30–32]. This should not affect the decision to start empiric antibiotics early in these patients.

2.6 Spinal column infections

Infections of the spinal column are an important diagnostic consideration in all patients presenting to the ED with back pain. Potential sources of infection in the spinal column include vertebral osteomyelitis, discitis, and epidural abscess. These infections are commonly missed, as there is remarkable variability in patient presentation and fever is seen in only half of these patients [33–35] Neurologic deficits likewise may or may not be present [33–35]. Risk factors for infections of the spinal column include immunocompromise, recent instrumentation, spinal implants, and use of intravenous drugs [35]. Magnetic resonance imaging (MRI) is the preferred imaging study in patients with suspected spinal column infection [35]. If MRI is unavailable, CT myelography can also be used [35].

2.7 Intraabdominal infections

Causes of intraabdominal sepsis include abdominal and pelvic abscesses, pelvic inflammatory disease, spontaneous bacterial peritonitis, cholecystitis or cholangitis, ruptured hollow viscus, or infection of the gastrointestinal tract. While abdominal sources for sepsis are common in the ED, the diagnosis may be hampered by examination difficulties secondary to the patient's mental status or body habitus. Altered consciousness can impede a patient's ability to localize their discomfort, and many abdominal pathologies have no manifestations on external visual examination. As such, a thorough abdominal examination is of vital importance in altered patients. Although these patients may be unable to verbalize discomfort, absent bowel sounds, abdominal distention, or abdominal rigidity on examination can be clues to the presence of intraabdominal pathology [36–38]. Additionally, grimacing, guarding, or reflex tachycardia can be useful indicators of pain in patients are altered or obtunded [36–38]. Pelvic examination should be done if a pelvic source is suspected or if there is concern for toxic shock syndrome secondary to a retained vaginal foreign body [38].

2.8 Indwelling devices

Indwelling devices such as urinary catheters, ports, pacers, and long-term intravenous access are associated with an increased risk of infection. Examination of these devices is an important part of the physical examination of the septic patient. Erythema or purulence at the exit site is specific for infection but these signs of not sensitive for the presence of device-associated infection. In fact, less than 5% of dialysis line-associated bacteremia was found to have associated purulent exit site drainage [39]. Because physical examination findings are often absent, it is important to keep device-associated infection in the differential in septic patients. If infection is suspected, the device should be removed as soon as clinically possible and cultured [39–41].

3. Hyperthermia

While a reflexive diagnosis of sepsis is tempting for the ill-appearing patient with an elevated temperature, it is important to consider conditions that mimic sepsis which are often both life-threatening and reversible. Unlike the fever associated with sepsis, the majority of these sepsis mimics have elevated temperature as a result of hyperthermia, which occurs secondary to dysfunction of the hypothalamic thermoregulatory system [1]. If an infectious source cannot be found in a seemingly septic patient or the patient is not improving with antibiotics and fluids, it is important to broaden the differential to conditions that cause hyperthermia (**Table 3**).

3.1 Neuroleptic malignant syndrome (NMS)

NMS is a life-threatening syndrome of altered mental status, autonomic instability, hyperthermia, and muscle rigidity associated with the use of dopaminergic antagonists. "Lead pipe" rigidity is the hallmark physical examination finding in NMS and can be severe enough to precipitate rhabdomyolysis. Most commonly, NMS occurs with the use of dopaminergic antagonists used in the treatment of psychiatric disorders and nausea, but NMS can also be precipitated by may be caused withdrawal from dopaminergic medications, such as those used in the treatment of Parkinson's disease [42, 43]. First generation antipsychotic medications are the most commonly implicated in NMS, with haloperidol and fluphenazine having the highest risk [42]. Risk factors for the development of NMS include higher medication doses, recent or rapid dose escalation, and parenteral medication administration [42].

Condition	Presentation	Management
Neuroleptic malignant syndrome	Delirium, hyperthermia, tachycardia, rigidity	Supportive, dantrolene sodium, bromocriptine
Serotonin syndrome	Delirium, hyperthermia, tachycardia, hyperreflexia/clonus.	Supportive, consider cyproheptadine
Malignant hyperthermia	Hyperthermia, tachycardia, hypercarbia, muscle rigidity in the setting of volatile anesthetic or depolarizing muscle relaxants	Dantrolene sodium, cooling measures, treatment of hyperkalemia
Salicylate toxicity	Delirium, hyperthermia, tachycardia, hyperpnea, gastrointestinal irritation, tinnitus, triple acid–base disturbance	Sodium bicarbonate
Anticholinergic toxicity	Delirium, tachycardia, dilated nonreactive pupils, urinary retention, anhidrotic hyperthermia	Supportive
Sympathomimetic toxicity or withdrawal from sympathetic antagonists	Delirium, tachycardia, hyperthermia, hypertension, dilated reactive pupils	Benzodiazepines
Thyroid storm	Tachycardia, hyperthermia, agitation, lid-lag, ophthalmopathy, hand tremor.	Beta-blocker, thionamide, steroids
Non-exertional heat stroke	Fever, tachycardia, neurologic manifestations	Evaporative and convective cooling

Table 3.
Hyperthermic sepsis mimics, their presentation, and their management.

The highest risk of NMS is within two weeks of medication initiation but this syndrome develop at any time during the treatment timeline [44]. A review of the patient's medications is typically needed to make the diagnosis. The cornerstone of management of NMS is supportive, with discontinuation of the suspected offending agent, support of the cardiopulmonary system, maintenance of normothermia and euvolemia, and prevention of complications including deep venous thrombosis, acute renal failure, and cardiac dysrhythmias [42–44]. In cases of severe muscle rigidity not responding to supportive treatment, intravenous dantrolene sodium or oral bromocriptine mesylate should be considered [44].

3.2 Serotonin syndrome (SS)

SS is a syndrome of altered mentation, neuromuscular abnormalities, and autonomic hyperactivity caused by excess serotonin levels [45]. The most commonly implicated medications in SS include linezolid, fentanyl, and selective serotonin reuptake inhibitor (SSRIs) [46]. The neuromuscular abnormalities associated with SS can include hyperreflexia, clonus, or muscle rigidity, and, as with NMS, these may be severe enough to which may lead to rhabdomyolysis [45, 46]. SS is a clinical diagnosis based on patient presentation, and there is no laboratory test or imaging study to confirm the diagnosis [45]. The Hunter criteria for serotonin syndrome is one outline the clinical criteria needed to make the diagnosis [47]. Like NMS, management of SS is primarily supportive. If this is insufficient or ineffective, use of cyproheptadine can be used under the consultation of a toxicologist [45]. If neuromuscular paralysis is need to control neuromuscular rigidity or facilitate intubation, only nondepolarizing agents should be used, as depolarizing agents may exacerbate the hyperkalemia precipitated by the neuromuscular abnormalities of SS [45, 46].

Spontaneous clonus
Inducible clonus AND agitation OR diaphoresis
Ocular clonus AND agitation OR diaphoresis
Tremor AND hyperreflexia
Hypertonia, temperature > 38°C AND ocular OR inducible clonus

Table 4.
Hunter criteria for serotonin syndrome [47].

Suspect serotonin syndrome if the patient has taken a serotonergic agent and has one of the symptom complexes outlined below (**Table 4**).

3.3 Malignant hyperthermia (MH)

MH is a genetic disorder which results in a hypermetabolic response to volatile anesthetics and depolarizing muscle relaxants [48]. This pathologic response to these medications results from caused the release of excessive calcium from the sarcoplasmic reticulum, which leads to uncoupling of oxidative phosphorylation, the release of heat, and a rise in metabolic rate [49]. MH presents with hyperthermia, tachycardia, hypercarbia, increased oxygen consumption, and muscle rigidity following the administration of a volatile anesthetic or depolarizing muscle relaxants. In the ED, MH is most likely to present following an intubation using succinylcholine and MH should be a diagnostic consideration in a patients with acute decompensation following intubation. MH is treated with intravenous dantrolene loaded at a dose of 2.5 mg/kg followed by boluses of 1 mg/kg until symptoms resolution [48]. Aggressive cardiopulmonary support, maintenance of normothermia and euvolemia, and treatment of electrolyte derangements is likewise important.

3.4 Salicylate toxicity

Aspirin ingestion is the most common cause of salicylate toxicity, but other common sources include Oil of Wintergreen, some wart removers, and keratolytics [50]. Salicylate toxicity is an important sepsis mimic, as patients with salicylate toxicity will have tachycardia, tachypnea, elevated temperature, and lactic acidosis. These symptoms occur secondary to salicylate interference with aerobic metabolism [50]. The classically described triad of salicylate toxicity is hyperpnea, tinnitus, and gastrointestinal irritation [51]. Gastrointestinal symptoms vary and can include abdominal pain, nausea, vomiting, and diarrhea. Tinnitus associated with salicylate toxicity may be described as hearing loss rather than "ringing in the ears" by patients and may be a difficult symptom to elicit if the patient is altered or obtunded [51]. Laboratory testing in salicylate toxicity will show a classic "triple acid-base disorder." This includes a respiratory alkalosis from hyperventilation, a compensatory non-gap metabolic acidosis, and an anion-gap metabolic acidosis from secondary to lactic acid accumulation [51]. Management is through systemic alkalinization with sodium bicarbonate [52].

3.5 Anticholinergic toxicity

Anticholinergic substances are ubiquitous in both pharmaceutical compounds and nature. Commonly encountered causes of anticholinergic toxicity include ingestion of antihistamine medications, tricyclic antidepressants, jimson weed, and tainted recreational drugs. Anticholinergic toxicity can easily be mistake for sepsis, as these patients present with high temperature, delirium, and tachycardia [53]. A distinguishing feature of anticholinergic toxicity is the presence of anhidrotic hyperthermia, in contrast to septic patients who are febrile and diaphoretic [53]. This is a result of anticholinergic blockade of sweat glands, preventing homeostatic hydrosis in response to elevated core temperature [53, 54]. Other clinical findings in anticholinergic toxicity include dry mucus membranes, dilated, non-reactive pupils and urinary retention [53]. The management of anticholinergic toxicity is primarily supportive. Benzodiazepines should be used for agitation or seizures [54]. Physostigmine, an anticholinesterase inhibitor, can be used as an antidote for anticholinergic toxicity under the consultation of a toxicologist [54].

3.6 Sympathomimetic toxicity or withdrawal from sympathetic antagonists

Overstimulation of the sympathetic nervous system can occur through direct agonism of the sympathetic receptors or withdrawal from substances that act as sympathetic antagonists [55]. Common sympathomimetic compounds encountered in the ED include cocaine, phencyclidine, and amphetamines. Withdrawal from alcohol or benzodiazepines can also result in sympathetic overstimulation [56]. Symptoms of sympathomimetic toxicity hyperthermia, tachycardia delirium, and reactive mydriasis [55]. Hyperthermia in sympathetic overstimulation results from direct agonism of alpha receptors as well as heat released by associated psychomotor agitation [55]. Benzodiazepines are mainstay of management of both sympathomimetic toxicity and withdrawal from antisympathetic agents [55].

3.7 Thyroid storm

Thyroid storm is the most severe manifestation of thyrotoxicosis and can be caused by overdose of therapeutic thyroid hormone or may present in patients with underlying thyrotoxicosis, seemingly unprovoked or may be precipitated by trauma, infection, childbirth, or other acute events [57]. Symptoms of thyroid storm include delirium, hyperthermia, diarrhea, and tachydysrhythmias, which can be severe enough to cause cardiovascular collapse and hemodynamic compromise [57, 58]. Liver failure may also occur [57]. The diagnostic laboratory abnormality in thyroid storm a severely low or undetectable thyroid stimulating hormone (TSH). Physical examination findings concerning for thyroid storm are those classically seen in hyperthyroidism and include ophthalmopathy, lid lag, thyromegaly, hand tremor, and global hyperreflexia [57, 58]. ED management of includes immediate treatment with a beta blocker, a thionamide, and glucocorticoids [59]. An iodine preparation should be given an hour after the administration of the thionamide, to prevent the iodine being used as substrate for the synthesis of more thyroid hormone [59]. If an infection is suspected as the cause of thyroid storm, broad-spectrum empiric antibiotics should be administered.

3.8 Heat stroke

Heat stroke is condition of elevated core body temperature with associated central nervous system dysfunction, commonly encephalopathy [60]. Heat stroke can be broadly divided into non-exertional and exertional. Non-exertional heat stroke classically affects older individuals with comorbidities that result in impaired thermoregulation, prevent access to adequate hydration, or inhibit removal from a hot environment [60]. In contrast, exertional heat stroke is more likely to occur in young, healthy individuals in the setting of exertion that overwhelms homeostatic thermoregulatory mechanisms. Heat stroke is a clinical diagnosis of exclusion made based on elevated body temperature (generally >40°C), central nervous system dysfunction (classically encephalopathy), and a history of exposure to severe environmental heat or excessive exertion [60]. Evaporative and convective cooling are the treatments of choice and should be initiated as soon as the diagnosis is made to improve morbidity and mortality [61, 62]. Common cooling methods used in the ED include ice water immersion, cooled fluid lavage, and evaporative cooling [61, 62]. In cases of refractory hyperthermia, dantrolene can be used as salvage therapy but its efficacy in this clinical context is uncertain [63, 64].

4. Conclusion

Elevated core temperature can be the result of either fever or hyperthermia. Fever is mor common and is typically caused by infections of the respiratory or urinary tracts. Other potential sources of infection include musculoskeletal, cardiac, neurological, and intra-abdominal as well as infection from indwelling medical devices. Treatment of patients with elevated core temperature should begin with fluids, empiric antimicrobials, and source control. If treatment of infection is ineffective or if the presentation is inconsistent with the presence of infection, the differential diagnosis should be expanded to consider conditions that cause hyperthermia as the cause of elevated core temperature. Such sepsis mimics include toxicity from medications and illicit substances, neuroleptic malignant syndrome, serotonin syndrome, malignant hyperthermia, thyroid storm, and heat stroke. Identification of these mimics as the source of elevated temperature leads to earlier diagnosis and improved prognosis in these patients.

Author details

Marina Boushra
The Respiratory Institute at the Cleveland Clinic, Cleveland, Ohio, United States of America

*Address all correspondence to: mnb9143@gmail.com

References

[1] Walter EJ, Hanna-Jumma S, Carraretto M, Forni L. The pathophysiological basis and consequences of fever. *Critical Care*. 2016;20(1):200. doi:10.1186/s13054-016-1375-5

[2] Bartfai T, Conti B. Fever. *The Scientific World Journal*. 2010;10:490-503. doi:10.1100/tsw.2010.50

[3] Kaul DR, Flanders SA, Beck JM, Saint S. Brief report: Incidence, etiology, risk factors, and outcome of hospital-acquired fever: A systematic, evidence-based review. *Journal of General Internal Medicine*. 2006;21(11):1184-1187. doi:10.1111/j.1525-1497.2006.00566.x

[4] Bor DH, Makadon HJ, Friedland G, Dasse P, Komaroff AL, Aronson MD. Fever in hospitalized medical patients - Characteristics and significance. *Journal of General Internal Medicine*. 1988;3(2):119-125. doi:10.1007/BF02596115

[5] Taeb AM, Hooper MH, Marik PE. Sepsis: Current Definition, Pathophysiology, Diagnosis, and Management. *Nutrition in Clinical Practice*. 2017;32(3):296-308. doi:10.1177/0884533617695243

[6] American College of Chest Physicians/Society of Critical Care Medicine Consensus Conference: definitions for sepsis and organ failure and guidelines for the use of innovative therapies in sepsis. *Critical care medicine*. 1992;20(6):864-874. http://www.ncbi.nlm.nih.gov/pubmed/1597042. Accessed February 10, 2018.

[7] Singer M, Deutschman CS, Seymour CW, et al. The Third International Consensus Definitions for Sepsis and Septic Shock (Sepsis-3). *JAMA*. 2016;315(8):801. doi:10.1001/jama.2016.0287

[8] Rhodes A, Evans LE, Alhazzani W, et al. Surviving Sepsis Campaign: International Guidelines for Management of Sepsis and Septic Shock: 2016. *Intensive Care Medicine*. 2017;43(3):304-377. doi:10.1007/s00134-017-4683-6

[9] Cavanaugh JB, Sullivan JB, East N, Nodzon JN. Importance of Pharmacy Involvement in the Treatment of Sepsis. *Hospital Pharmacy*. 2017;52(3):191-197. doi:10.1310/hpj5203-191

[10] Moussavi K, Nikitenko V. Pharmacist impact on time to antibiotic administration in patients with sepsis in an ED. *The American Journal of Emergency Medicine*. 2016;34(11):2117-2121. doi:10.1016/j.ajem.2016.07.031

[11] Laine ME, Flynn JD, Flannery AH. Impact of Pharmacist Intervention on Selection and Timing of Appropriate Antimicrobial Therapy in Septic Shock. *Journal of Pharmacy Practice*. 2018;31(1):46-51. doi:10.1177/0897190017696953

[12] Gastmeier P, Kampf G, Wischnewski N, ... TH-J of H, 1998 undefined. Prevalence of nosocomial infections in representative German hospitals. *Elsevier*. https://www.sciencedirect.com/science/article/pii/S0195670198901736. Accessed October 13, 2020.

[13] Jain S, Self WH, Wunderink RG, et al. Community-Acquired Pneumonia Requiring Hospitalization among U.S. Adults. *The New England journal of medicine*. 2015;373(5):415-427. doi:10.1056/NEJMoa1500245

[14] Cillóniz C, Ewig S, Polverino E, et al. Microbial aetiology of community-acquired pneumonia and its relation to severity. *Thorax*. 2011;66(4):340-346. doi:10.1136/thx.2010.143982

[15] Ewig S, Welte T, Torres A. Is healthcare-associated pneumonia a distinct entity needing specific therapy? *Current opinion in infectious diseases*. 2012;25(2):166-175. doi:10.1097/QCO.0b013e32835023fb

[16] Johansen T, Cek M, Naber K, urology LS-E, 2007 undefined. Prevalence of hospital-acquired urinary tract infections in urology departments. *Elsevier*. https://www.sciencedirect.com/science/article/pii/S0302283806009365?casa_token=tx0EZL4s2ZoAAAAA:VUDyuCMPljmzF4xbstHRc1xuxmHJLjso3z8qabxrdz-BaDrAfN9Fqx3tsL1q5AlUqrpHyLLl_qU. Accessed October 13, 2020.

[17] Kalra O. Approach to a patient with urosepsis. *Journal of Global Infectious Diseases*. 2009;1(1):57. doi:10.4103/0974-777x.52984

[18] Stamm WE, Hooton TM, Hooton TM. Management of urinary tract infections in adults. *The New England journal of medicine*. 1993;329(18):1328-1334. doi:10.1056/NEJM199310283291808

[19] Nicolle LE, AMMI Canada Guidelines Committee* ACG. Complicated urinary tract infection in adults. *The Canadian journal of infectious diseases & medical microbiology = Journal canadien des maladies infectieuses et de la microbiologie medicale*. 2005;16(6):349-360. http://www.ncbi.nlm.nih.gov/pubmed/18159518. Accessed December 16, 2016

[20] Stevens DL, Bisno AL, Chambers HF, et al. Practice guidelines for the diagnosis and management of skin and soft tissue infections: 2014 update by the infectious diseases society of America. *Clinical Infectious Diseases*. 2014;59(2). doi:10.1093/cid/ciu296

[21] Horowitz DL, Katzap E, Horowitz S, Barilla-LaBarca M-L. Approach to septic arthritis. *American family physician*. 2011;84(6):653-660. http://www.ncbi.nlm.nih.gov/pubmed/21916390. Accessed February 13, 2018.

[22] Hassan AS, Rao A, Manadan AM, Block JA. Peripheral Bacterial Septic Arthritis: Review of Diagnosis and Management. *Jcr: Journal of Clinical Rheumatology*. 2017;23(8):435-442. doi:10.1097/rhu.0000000000000588

[23] Htwe TH, Khardori NM. Cardiac emergencies: Infective endocarditis, pericarditis, and myocarditis. *Medical Clinics of North America*. 2012;96(6):1149-1169. doi:10.1016/j.mcna.2012.09.003

[24] Lange RA, Hillis LD. Acute Pericarditis. *New England Journal of Medicine*. 2004;351(21):2195-2202. doi:10.1056/NEJMcp041997

[25] Cahill TJ, Prendergast BD. Infective endocarditis. *Lancet (London, England)*. 2016;387(10021):882-893. doi:10.1016/S0140-6736(15)00067-7

[26] Tunkel AR, Hartman BJ, Kaplan SL, et al. Practice Guidelines for the Management of Bacterial Meningitis. *Clinical Infectious Diseases*. 2004;39(9):1267-1284. doi:10.1086/425368

[27] Brouwer MC, Tunkel AR, van de Beek D. Epidemiology, diagnosis, and antimicrobial treatment of acute bacterial meningitis. *Clinical microbiology reviews*. 2010;23(3):467-492. doi:10.1128/CMR.00070-09

[28] Logan SAE, MacMahon E. Viral meningitis. *BMJ*. 2008;336(7634):36-40. doi:10.1136/BMJ.39409.673657.AE

[29] Lucas S. Acute bacterial meningitis during and after pregnancy. *BJOG: An International Journal of Obstetrics & Gynaecology*. 2012;119(13):1555-1557. doi:10.1111/1471-0528.12025

[30] Blazer S, Berant M, Alon U. Bacterial meningitis. Effect of antibiotic treatment on cerebrospinal fluid. *American journal of clinical pathology*. 1983;80(3):386-387. http://www.ncbi.nlm.nih.gov/pubmed/6881104. Accessed February 10, 2018.

[31] Nigrovic LE, Malley R, Macias CG, et al. Effect of antibiotic pretreatment on cerebrospinal fluid profiles of children with bacterial meningitis. *Pediatrics*. 2008;122(4):726-730. doi:10.1542/peds.2007-3275

[32] Kanegaye JT, Soliemanzadeh P, Bradley JS. Lumbar puncture in pediatric bacterial meningitis: defining the time interval for recovery of cerebrospinal fluid pathogens after parenteral antibiotic pretreatment. *Pediatrics*. 2001;108(5):1169-1174. http://www.ncbi.nlm.nih.gov/pubmed/11694698. Accessed February 10, 2018.

[33] Torda AJ, Gottlieb T, Bradbury R. Pyogenic vertebral osteomyelitis: analysis of 20 cases and review. *Clinical infectious diseases : an official publication of the Infectious Diseases Society of America*. 1995;20(2):320-328. http://www.ncbi.nlm.nih.gov/pubmed/7742437. Accessed February 10, 2018.

[34] Sapico FL, Montgomerie JZ. Pyogenic vertebral osteomyelitis: report of nine cases and review of the literature. *Reviews of infectious diseases*. 1(5):754-776. http://www.ncbi.nlm.nih.gov/pubmed/542761. Accessed February 10, 2018.

[35] Berbari EF, Kanj SS, Kowalski TJ, et al. 2015 Infectious Diseases Society of America (IDSA) Clinical Practice Guidelines for the Diagnosis and Treatment of Native Vertebral Osteomyelitis in Adults. *Clinical infectious diseases : an official publication of the Infectious Diseases Society of America*. 2015;61(6):e26-46. doi:10.1093/cid/civ482

[36] Solomkin JS, Mazuski JE, Bradley JS, et al. Diagnosis and Management of Complicated Intra-abdominal Infection in Adults and Children: Guidelines by the Surgical Infection Society and the Infectious Diseases Society of America. *Clinical Infectious Diseases*. 2010;50(2):133-164. doi:10.1086/649554

[37] Swenson RM, Lorber B, Michaelson TC, Spaulding EH. The Bacteriology of Intra-abdominal Infections. *Archives of Surgery*. 1974;109(3):398. doi:10.1001/archsurg.1974.01360030050013

[38] Walker CK, Wiesenfeld HC. Antibiotic Therapy for Acute Pelvic Inflammatory Disease: The 2006 Centers for Disease Control and Prevention Sexually Transmitted Diseases Treatment Guidelines. *Clinical Infectious Diseases*. 2007;44(Supplement 3):S111-S122. doi:10.1086/511424

[39] Troidle L, Finkelstein FO. Catheter-related bacteremia in hemodialysis patients: the role of the central venous catheter in prevention and therapy. *The International journal of artificial organs*. 2008;31(9):827-833. http://www.ncbi.nlm.nih.gov/pubmed/18924095. Accessed February 11, 2018.

[40] Sychev D, Maya ID, Allon M. Clinical Management of Dialysis Catheter-Related Bacteremia with Concurrent Exit-Site Infection. *Seminars in Dialysis*. 2011;24(2):239-241. doi:10.1111/j.1525-139X.2011.00869.x

[41] Ramanathan V, Darouiche RO. Prevention and management of hemodialysis catheter infections. *Expert Review of Anti-infective Therapy*. 2012;10(12):1447-1455. doi:10.1586/eri.12.134

[42] Adnet P, Lestavel P, Krivosic-Horber R. Neuroleptic malignant syndrome. *British Journal of Anaesthesia*. 2000;85(1):129-135. doi:10.1093/bja/85.1.129

[43] Bond W. Detection and Management of Neuroleptic Malignant Syndrome. *Clinical pharmacology*. 1984;3(302).

[44] Reulbach U, Dütsch C, Biermann T, et al. Managing an effective treatment for neuroleptic malignant syndrome. *Critical Care*. 2007;11(1):R4. doi:10.1186/cc5148

[45] Boyer EW, Shannon M. The Serotonin Syndrome. *New England Journal of Medicine*. 2005;352(11): 1112-1120. doi:10.1056/NEJMra041867

[46] Ables AZ, Nagubilli R. Prevention, recognition, and management of serotonin syndrome. *American family physician*. 2010;81(9):1139-1142. http://www.ncbi.nlm.nih.gov/pubmed/20433130. Accessed February 11, 2018.

[47] Dunkley EJC, Isbister GK, Sibbritt D, Dawson AH, Whyte IM. The Hunter Serotonin Toxicity Criteria: simple and accurate diagnostic decision rules for serotonin toxicity. *QJM : monthly journal of the Association of Physicians*. 2003;96(9):635-642. http://www.ncbi.nlm.nih.gov/pubmed/12925718. Accessed February 11, 2018.

[48] Glahn KPE, Ellis FR, Halsall PJ, et al. Recognizing and managing a malignant hyperthermia crisis: guidelines from the European Malignant Hyperthermia Group. *British Journal of Anaesthesia*. 2010;105(4):417-420. doi:10.1093/bja/aeq243

[49] Rosenberg H, Pollock N, Schiemann A, Bulger T, Stowell K. Malignant hyperthermia: a review. *Orphanet Journal of Rare Diseases*. 2015;10. doi:10.1186/S13023-015-0310-1

[50] O'Malley GF. Emergency Department Management of the Salicylate-Poisoned Patient. *Emergency Medicine Clinics*. 2007;25(2):333-346. doi:10.1016/J.EMC.2007.02.012

[51] Bari N. Salicylate poisoning. *JPMA The Journal of the Pakistan Medical Association*. 1995;45(6):160-161. http://www.ncbi.nlm.nih.gov/pubmed/7474293. Accessed February 11, 2018.

[52] Chyka PA, Erdman AR, Christianson G, et al. Salicylate poisoning: An evidence-based consensus guideline for out-of-hospital management. *Clinical Toxicology*. 2007;45(2):95-131. doi:10.1080/15563650600907140

[53] Dawson AH, Buckley NA. Pharmacological management of anticholinergic delirium - theory, evidence and practice. *British journal of clinical pharmacology*. 2016;81(3): 516-524. doi:10.1111/bcp.12839

[54] Oakley P. Physostigmine versus diazepines for anticholinergic poisoning. *Annals of emergency medicine*. 2001;37(2):239-241. http://www.ncbi.nlm.nih.gov/pubmed/11174251. Accessed February 11, 2018.

[55] Hayes BD, Martinez JP, Barrueto F. Drug-induced hyperthermic syndromes. Part I. Hyperthermia in overdose. *Emergency Medicine Clinics of North America*. 2013;31(4):1019-1033. doi:10.1016/j.emc.2013.07.004

[56] Paden MS, Franjic L, Halcomb SE. Hyperthermia caused by drug interactions and adverse reactions. *Emergency Medicine Clinics of North America*. 2013;31(4):1035-1044. doi:10.1016/j.emc.2013.07.003

[57] Chiha M, Samarasinghe S, Kabaker AS. Thyroid Storm. *Journal of Intensive Care Medicine*. 2015;30(3): 131-140. doi:10.1177/0885066613498053

[58] Nayak B, Burman K. Thyrotoxicosis and Thyroid Storm. doi:10.1016/j.ecl.2006.09.008

[59] Ross DS, Burch HB, Cooper DS, et al. 2016 American Thyroid

Association Guidelines for Diagnosis and Management of Hyperthyroidism and Other Causes of Thyrotoxicosis. *Thyroid*. 2016;26(10):1343-1421. doi:10.1089/thy.2016.0229

[60] Yeo TP. Heat stroke: a comprehensive review. *AACN clinical issues*. 15(2):280-293. http://www.ncbi.nlm.nih.gov/pubmed/15461044. Accessed February 11, 2018.

[61] Smith JE, Wallis L. Cooling methods used in the treatment of exertional heat illness. *British journal of sports medicine*. 2005;39(8):503-507; discussion 507. doi:10.1136/bjsm.2004.013466

[62] Gaudio FG, Grissom CK. Cooling Methods in Heat Stroke. *The Journal of Emergency Medicine*. 2016;50(4):607-616. doi:10.1016/j.jemermed.2015.09.014

[63] Moran D, Epstein Y, Wiener M, Horowitz M. Dantrolene and recovery from heat stroke. *Aviation, space, and environmental medicine*. 1999;70(10):987-989. http://www.ncbi.nlm.nih.gov/pubmed/10519477. Accessed February 11, 2018.

[64] Hadad E, Cohen-Sivan Y, Heled Y, Epstein Y. Clinical review: Treatment of heat stroke: should dantrolene be considered? *Critical Care*. 2004;9(1):86. doi:10.1186/cc2923

Section 2

Damage Control Surgery and Liver Trauma

Chapter 3

Damage Control Surgery for Liver Trauma

Ioannis A. Ziogas, Ioannis Katsaros and Georgios Tsoulfas

Abstract

The liver is one of the most commonly injured organs of the abdomen after major trauma and may lead to the extravasation of major amounts of blood. Damage control surgery (DCS) as a concept exists for over one hundred years but has been more widely optimized and implemented over the past few decades. Minimizing the time from the trauma scene to the hospital and recognizing the patterns of injury and the "lethal triad" (acidosis, hypothermia, coagulopathy) is vital to understand which patients will benefit the most from DCS. Immediate patient resuscitation, massive blood transfusion, and taking the patient to the operating room as soon as possible are the critical initial steps that have been associated with improved outcomes. Bleeding and contamination control should be the priority in this first exploratory laparotomy, while the patient should be transferred to the intensive care unit postoperatively with only temporary abdominal wall closure. Once the patient is stabilized, a second operation should be performed where an anatomic liver resection or other more major procedures may take place, along with permanent closure of the abdominal wall.

Keywords: liver trauma, hypothermia, acidosis, coagulopathy, perihepatic packing

1. Introduction

Despite its well-protected position, the liver is the most frequently affected abdominal organ by blunt or penetrating trauma [1, 2]. Over the past decades, the improvements in the assessment and management of hepatic injury have evolved significantly, thus resulting in better outcomes for affected patients [3]. The majority of such injuries develop following high-energy traffic accidents or violent behaviors [4]. Industrial and farming accidents also consist of a significant percentage of liver trauma. Blunt injuries are the majority of cases in Europe, Australia, and Asia, whereas penetrating injuries (stab and gunshot wounds) are most frequently encountered in North America and South Africa [5, 6].

Blunt trauma, as a result of traffic accident or fall from a height, may lead to deceleration injury due to the inertia of the liver [4]. The affected sites usually involve the attachments to the diaphragm and abdominal wall. These types of injury typically involve the right lobe, especially the posterior segments, and the caudate lobe, while a vascular injury may also be present with the respective hepatic arteries, portal and hepatic veins being affected [4, 7, 8]. The site of connection between inferior vena cava and hepatic veins is vulnerable to blunt traumas and may lead to serious venous injuries and a significant blood loss. Penetrating injuries are more frequently associated with significant vascular injuries at the liver site inflicted [4].

 IntechOpen

In this chapter, we aimed to describe the classification and appropriate investigations of liver injuries and elaborate on the use of damage control surgery (DCS) in this setting.

2. Liver anatomy

The liver is a wedge-shaped abdominal organ and is located in the right hypochondrium and epigastrium and may extend into the left hypochondrium [9, 10]. It is covered by fibrous Glisson's capsule and is attached to the surrounding structures and the abdominal wall by several ligaments (falciform, coronary, triangular, hepatoduodenal and hepatogastric ligaments). It is divided into two lobes (right and left) by the falciform ligament, while two "accessory" lobes, the caudate and quadrate lobe, arise from the right lobe. The liver has unique double blood supply from the proper hepatic artery (25%) and portal vein (75%). Venous drainage is achieved through hepatic veins (right, middle, left) to the inferior vena cava.

3. Liver functional anatomy – Couinaud classification system

The Couinaud classification is the most widely used classification for functional liver anatomy [11]. It divides the liver into eight functionally independent segments, which have their own individual vascular supply and biliary drainage (**Figure 1**) [12]. A branch of the portal vein, hepatic artery, and bile duct are centrally located in each segment, while the vascular outflow to hepatic veins is located peripherally. Due to their functional independence, each segment can be safely resected without damaging the remaining liver parenchyma [13]. Nevertheless, the Couinaud classification system does not take into account the influence of vascular variations and does not provide liver surface landmarks for segment separation [14].

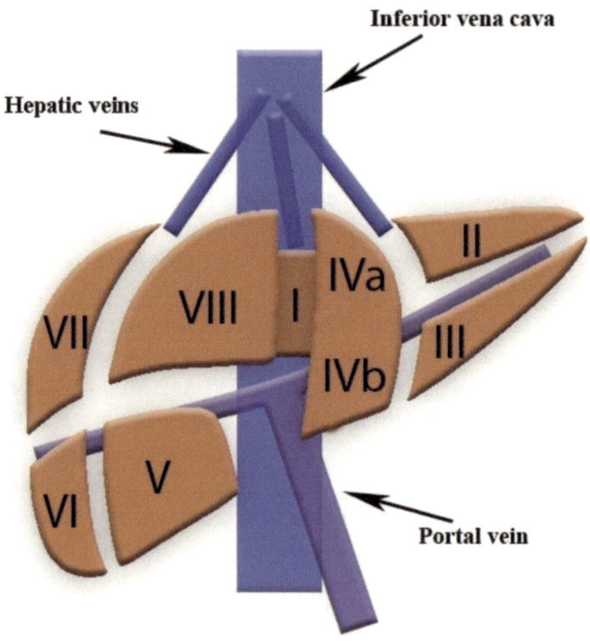

Figure 1.
Liver functional anatomy – Couinaud classification system.

The liver segments are divided by portal vein branches and hepatic veins and are numbered clockwise [12]. The portal vein bifurcates at hepatic hilum into the left and right branches, which separate the liver into upper and lower segments. The right and left lobes are divided by middle hepatic vein, which runs along the Cantlie's line from the inferior vena cava to the gallbladder fossa [15] Furthermore, the right hepatic vein divides the right lobe into anterior and posterior segments and left hepatic vein divides the left lobe into medial and lateral parts.

The Caudate lobe (segment 1) is located posteriorly and often drains directly to inferior vena cava, while it can be supplied by both the right and the left portal vein branches, while segments II (superiorly) and III (inferiorly) are located medial to the left hepatic vein [16]. Segment IV (quadrate lobe) is located between the left and middle hepatic veins and is further divided by Bismuth into IVa (superiorly) and IVb (inferiorly) [17]. The anterior segments of the right hemiliver, V (inferiorly) and VIII (superiorly) lie between the middle and right hepatic veins, while the posterior right hemiliver segments, VI (inferiorly) and VII (superiorly), are located lateral to the right hepatic vein.

4. Liver trauma classification

The American Association for the Surgery of Trauma (AAST) grading scale is widely utilized for the classification of liver injury severity (**Table 1**) [18, 19]. However, it does not take into consideration the hemodynamic status of patients and the associated injuries. Thus, the World Society of Emergency Surgery (WSES) proposed a novel classification for the proper management of hepatic injuries involving AAST grade (1994 revision), hemodynamic stability, and mechanism of injury (**Table 2**) [2, 20].

Minor (WSES grade I) and moderate (WSES grade II) liver injuries concern hemodynamically stable patients after either blunt or penetrating trauma with AAST grade I-II or III lesions, respectively. Severe hepatic injuries include

AAST grade	Injury description
I	Subcapsular hematoma <10% of surface
	Parenchymal laceration or capsular tear <1 cm depth
II	Subcapsular hematoma 10–50% of surface area; intraparenchymal hematoma, <10 cm diameter
	Parenchymal laceration 1–3 cm in depth or < 10 cm in length
III	Subcapsular hematoma >50% of surface area or expanding; ruptured subcapsular or parenchymal hematoma; intraparenchymal hematoma >10 cm in diameter
	Parenchymal laceration >3 cm in depth
	Any liver vascular injury or active bleeding contained within liver parenchyma
IV	Parenchymal disruption 25–75% of hepatic lobe
	Active bleeding extending beyond the liver parenchyma into the peritoneum
V	Parenchymal disruption >75% of hepatic lobe
	Juxtahepatic venous injury including retroheaptic vena cava and major hepatic veins

Grade is based on highest grade assessment made during imaging, intraoperatively or pathologic specimen. Advance one grade for multiple injuries up to grade III.

Table 1.
The American Association for the Surgery of Trauma (AAST) liver injury scale (2018 revision).

	WSES grade	AAST grade*	Mechanism of Injury	Hemodynamic status	CT-scan	First-line treatment
MINOR	I	I-II	Blunt/penetrating	Stable	YES + local exploration in stab wounds	NOM + clinical/laboratory/radiological evaluation
MODERATE	II	III	Blunt/penetrating	Stable		
SEVERE	III	IV-V	Blunt/penetrating	Stable		
	IV	I-VI	Blunt/penetrating	Unstable	NO	Surgery

NOM: non-operative management.

**American Association for the Surgery of Trauma (AAST) liver injury scale (1994 revision).*

Table 2.
The World Society of Emergency Surgery (WSES) classification and management of liver trauma.

hemodynamically stable, AAST grade IV-VI lesions following penetrating or blunt trauma (WSES grade III) (**Figure 2**) or any hemodynamically unstable lesion (WSES grade IV).

The importance of the WSES classification and management approach is highlighted by the fact that patients suffering from high-grade AAST lesions, which are hemodynamically stable, can be successfully treated non-operatively [21]. On the contrary, "minor" AAST injuries combined with hemodynamic instability must be treated operatively in order to control the intrabdominal bleeding [20].

5. Initial assessment and investigation

A liver injury should always be suspected in all patients suffering from a blunt or penetrating thoracoabdominal trauma, especially at the right site. Initial management of these patients should be based on the Advanced Trauma Life Support (ATLS) guidelines with fluid resuscitation and close monitoring being the first priorities [22]. Depending on the underlying injury mechanism, other concurrent injuries should also be evaluated and treated accordingly. The management of multi-trauma patients should take into consideration all the affected organs, and a multidisciplinary team is essential for the optimal treatment approach of these patients.

As far as hepatic trauma is concerned, in hemodynamically unstable patients, despite adequate fluid resuscitation, an immediate operation for bleeding control is indicated, whereas in stable patients, an appropriate workup protocol using ultrasonography or computerized tomography scanning (CT) can be followed. Hemodynamic instability is characterized by the following: heart rate > 120 bpm, systolic blood pressure < 90 mmHg, low urine output, increased respiratory rate (>30 respirations/minute), signs of skin vasoconstriction and altered level of consciousness [22]. Non-operative management necessitates medical centers capable of an accurate injury severity diagnosis, intensive management of patients, and prompt access to diagnostic modalities, interventional radiology, operation theater, and blood–blood products [20, 23].

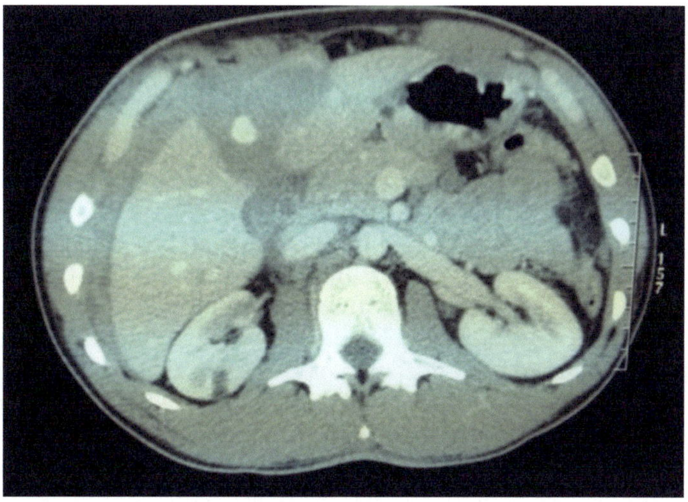

Figure 2.
Computed tomography scan demonstrating a severe liver injury.

Ultrasound plays a significant role in the proper investigation of abdominal injuries. Focused Assessment with Sonography for Trauma (FAST) can be performed immediately at the emergency department and can help assess the pericardium, hepatorenal space (Morison's pouch), perisplenic space and Douglas pouch to identify the presence of free fluid [22]. More detailed ultrasonography by an experienced radiologist is necessary for a more accurate investigation of liver parenchyma. Ultrasonography has widely replaced diagnostic peritoneal lavage (DPL) and has a high specificity of 95–100% [24]. Nevertheless, ultrasound examination is highly operator-depended and should be performed by experienced clinicians.

Computerized tomography (CT) scan is a valuable tool for the evaluation of stable patients with an abdominal injury [25]. A contrast-enhanced, multi-slice CT scan is reported to have a sensitivity and specificity of over 95% for detecting liver injuries [26, 27]. Subscapular and intraparenchymal hematomas, lacerations, and vascular injuries can be recognized. Furthermore, an active hemorrhage can be visualized as an extravasation of contrast medium. A CT scan can also successfully elucidate other abdominal injuries involving the spleen, kidneys, and bowel [26]. Finally, a follow-up CT scan can be utilized for the detection of delayed liver injury complications, including delayed hemorrhage, bile leak, biloma, arteriovenous malformations, and liver abscesses [4, 28].

6. Damage control surgery - general

Damage control surgery refers to the immediate steps taken in order to reduce blood loss, the risk of sepsis, morbidity, and mortality instead of a thorough patient workup in the intensive care unit (ICU) [29]. DCS has significantly improved the outcomes of patients presenting at the hospital with severe organ injuries, including liver injuries, and hemodynamic instability due to maneuvers to control the bleeding [1]. Uncontrolled bleeding can lead to coagulopathy secondary to the dilution and depletion of the coagulation factors, hypothermia, and acidosis, the so-called "lethal triad" or "medical bleeding" [21]. The onset of this series of events may necessitate the need for DCS, including temporary (perihepatic) packing of the bleeding sites, where physiological recovery is prioritized over anatomical repair [30].

7. Damage control surgery – history

The earliest report on perihepatic packing to prevent uncontrolled bleeding from injuries to the liver dates back to 1908 by James Pringle [31], while later in 1913, Halstead described the use of a rubber sheet between the injured liver and the gauze packs [32]. Despite the improvements in outcomes, perihepatic packing was sparsely described in the literature [33] until Stone et al. [34] reported a survival rate of 76% in patients managed with "truncated laparotomy" compared to 7% in patients managed with definitive surgical repair. Rotondo et al. [35] introduced the term "damage control laparotomy" and demonstrated that this approach could improve survival in hemorrhaging trauma patients (requiring transfusion of >10 units of packed red blood cells) with multiple visceral penetrating injuries and major vessel injuries. The authors described the three steps of their approach, and the same research group later modified it by introducing a fourth pre-operative phase (**Table 3**) [36]. Since then, DCS has been successfully implemented for the management of major liver injury with optimal outcomes. The use of angioembolization in more recent series has been proposed as the logical augmentation

Damage control (DC) Phase	Description
DC0	• Truncated scene times • Recognition of injury pattern • Immediate blood component replacement • Rewarming maneuvers
DCI	• Once in the operating room • Immediate exploratory laparotomy • Rapid bleeding and contamination control • Abdominal packing • Temporary wound closure
DCII	• Once in the intensive care unit • Physiological and biochemical stabilization • Thorough tertiary examination to identify all injuries
DCIII	• Once physiology is normalized • Re-exploration in operating room • Definitive repair of all injuries • May require multiple visits to the operating room if multiple systems are injured

Table 3.
The four Phases of damage control for exsanguinating penetrating abdominal injury by Johnson et al.

of damage control approaches to control bleeding, but particularly in the case of high-grade injuries, it may lead to major hepatic necrosis [37].

8. Damage control surgery – indications

As mentioned earlier, DCS can play a vital role in the setting of the "lethal triad" and thus metabolic acidosis (pH <7.2), hypothermia (<34°C), and coagulopathy (prolonged activated partial thromboplastin time and prothrombin time > two times normal) constitute absolute indications for DCS. Uncontrolled major intra-abdominal bleeding, association with extra-abdominal injury, >10 units of blood transfusion, and hemodynamic instability (low blood pressure and tachycardia) are relative indications for DCS [29].

9. Damage control surgery – phases

9.1 Damage control phase 0 (DC0)

DC0 constitutes the first phase of the DCS process and takes place in the pre-hospital setting and in the emergency room. The most crucial aspects of this phase are injury pattern recognition in order to determine which patients will most likely benefit from DCS according to the absolute and relative indications, and the "scoop and run" concept to truncate scene times. The administration of blood products and tranexamic acid in the pre-hospital setting has been increasingly used [38, 39]. Given the significant improvements in trauma resuscitation strategies aiming at rapid bleeding control, management of coagulopathy, and diversion away from the over-resuscitation with crystalloids, the use of DCS may be required to a lesser extent in the future [40–42]. There is a growing body of evidence that the use of a high plasma to packed red blood cell ratio can lead to a decrease in hemorrhage-related mortality [43]. French lyophilized plasma – manufactured by the French Military

Blood Institute – is a universal therapeutic viro-inactivated plasma that can be reconstituted in <6 min at the point-of-care and is compatible with any blood type [44]. Data suggest that French lyophilized plasma can be used more rapidly correct for the trauma-induced coagulopathy compared to fresh frozen plasma, particularly in the military setting [45]. Its role against normal saline in the management of post-traumatic coagulopathy prevention and correction in the pre-hospital civilian setting is currently under investigation (PREHO-PLYO study) [46], and it is awaited to revolutionize the current state of practice for the management of severe trauma, including liver injury.

Once the patients reach the emergency room, immediate assessment by the trauma team and damage control resuscitation is vital. The surgical and critical care teams should strive towards obtaining vascular access with two large-bore catheters, inserting nasogastric tube and urinary catheter (unless there is blood at the urethral meatus, high riding prostate or prevalent perineal hematoma), rapid induction of anesthesia, drainage of the chest (if needed), intravenous broad-spectrum antibiotics and tetanus prophylaxis (if indicated), rapid rewarming and prevention of further hypothermia, and expedited transport to the operating room for DCS [30].

9.2 Damage control phase I (DCI)

DCI starts with the exploratory laparotomy, which aims to control bleeding and limit contamination, and ends with the temporary closure of the abdominal wall. After the patient is positioned in a "cruciform" lie, the patient is prepped from chin to mid-thighs and a vertical midline incision from the xiphoid process to the pubic symphysis is made [30]. If the suspicion for a severe fracture of the pelvis is high, the incision should be limited just below the umbilicus to facilitate continuous tamponade of the suspected pelvic hematoma. If the patient is unstable, the incision should not be delayed if arterial or venous lines are not in place; these can be inserted during the operation.

If the observed intra-abdominal bleeding is not considered to be major, compression on its own or the use of topical hemostatic agents, bipolar devices or electrocautery, argon beam coagulation, omental patching or even simple suturing of the liver parenchyma may be adequate to control the hemorrhage [2, 20, 47–49]. In the case of massive intra-abdominal hemorrhage, more aggressive maneuvers should be adopted, including perihepatic packing and manual compression, or even hepatic vascular isolation (i.e., intrahepatic balloon tamponade) [50, 51]. Injuries to the portal vein should be primarily repaired, while ligation of the portal vein should be considered only as an alternative – provided that the proper hepatic artery is intact – due to the increased risk of hepatic necrosis or massive intestinal edema [47]. Data suggest preferring liver packing or resection over portal vein ligation if only lobar or segmental branches of the portal vein are injured [2, 47, 52]. However, portal vein ligation is safer than arterial ligation regarding biliary complications or hepatic necrosis, and may even prepare the liver for staged extended liver resection [53]. If the surgeon comes across a proper hepatic artery injury, they should shoot for a primary repair; otherwise, selective hepatic artery ligation should be preferred, and if the common or right hepatic artery is to be ligated, cholecystectomy should follow to prevent gallbladder necrosis [1, 52]. When arterial control or the Pringle maneuver is inadequate to control the hemorrhage, the surgeon should suspect that there might be an aberrant hepatic artery [47]. If the bleeding arises from the area behind the liver, the injury is most likely to be found on the hepatic or retro-hepatic caval vein [2, 47, 54]. Inserting vascular shunts (i.e., atrio-caval shunt) might also be useful to control hemorrhage [29, 47]. In case of persistent bleeding and hemodynamic instability, resuscitative endovascular balloon occlusion of the aorta in the zone I and of the vena cava at the level of the retro-hepatic vena cava can serve as a bridge to more definitive procedures [47]. Liver resection should be avoided at this phase, but if absolutely necessary, non-anatomic resections should be preferred [2, 47, 48, 52], while resection of a hemorrhaging spleen or kidney can be performed, if needed in order to stop the bleeding [29]. Angioembolization should be advocated for either stable patients after the initial surgical hemostatic attempt or adjunctively in case of suspected uncontrolled bleeding despite the surgical hemostatic attempt [2, 47, 55]; data also suggest that its routine implementation immediately after DCS can significantly improve survival in grade IV or V liver injury [56]. Regarding contamination control, intrahepatic abscesses can be managed with percutaneous drainage, and bilomas may either resolve spontaneously or should also be managed with percutaneous drainage potentially with adjunct therapeutic endoscopic retrograde cholangiopancreatography and stent placement [47]. Abdominal wall closure is the final step before transitioning to DCII (transfer to the ICU) and should be only temporary without fascial closure to avoid abdominal compartment syndrome [30].

9.3 Damage control phase II (DCII)

DCII involves taking the patient to the ICU postoperatively, where the goal is to restore the biochemical and physiological derangements. Managing fluid administration to bring the patient back to hemodynamic stability is often achieved through invasive monitoring (i.e., transthoracic echocardiography, transesophageal Doppler, pulmonary artery catheterization, etc.) [30]. Securing adequate oxygenation and aggressive rewarming of the patient are also necessary. The management of coagulopathy is crucial for survival, and the use of rotational thromboelastometry and other tests to assess how the coagulation cascade works along with massive blood transfusion practices have led to an improvement in outcomes and a decrease in blood transfusion requirements [30, 57]. Prevention of potentially fatal complications commonly seen in the ICU, including infection, adult respiratory distress syndrome, and deep vein thrombosis, is also important for patient survival [29]. This is the perfect opportunity for treating physicians to perform a complete reassessment of the patient and a "tertiary survey", including imaging studies that may help identify previously unknown injuries.

9.4 Damage control phase III (DCIII)

DCIII involves definite repair of the injuries once the patient is stabilized and has returned to his "physiologic normality" and commonly takes place within 24–72 hours after admission to the ICU. The patient is taken back to the operating room for re-exploration and packing removal (preferably after 48 hours) [21]. That is also the stage when an anatomic liver resection may be performed (**Figure 3**), along with the removal of devitalized tissue or vascular shunts, anastomosis of vessels or bowel, or even a feeding jejunostomy. The phase ends with the permanent closure of the abdominal wall. This should be performed with the approximation of the fascial edges if gentle adduction permits; if this is not possible due to retroperitoneal or bowel wall edema, then the abdominal wall should be again only temporarily closed with the fascia left open. In that scenario, the patient is taken back to the ICU and provided the patient is hemodynamically stable, administration of diuretics to decrease the bowel edema should be considered [30]. This situation should then be managed with washouts and re-inspection of the abdomen regularly, while primary closure should be completed within seven days, particularly in the absence of signs

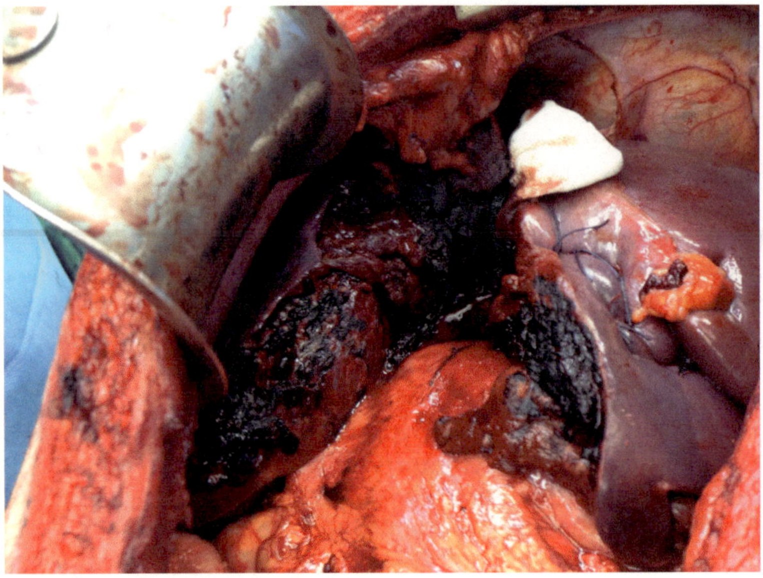

Figure 3.
Surgical management of severe liver injury with active bleeding.

of infection. Other abdominal closure alternatives should be considered if this is not possible. This will lead to a large ventral hernia that will require repair at some future time point [30].

10. Conclusion

Immediate resuscitation and DCS play a critical role in the outcomes of trauma patients in general, and particularly in those with severe liver injuries where the exsanguination of large amounts of blood is common. The decrease in the time from the scene to hospital and taking, the implementation of massive transfusion protocols, and the improvements in the approaches to control bleeding and contamination intraoperatively by leaving major resections for a later phase have revolutionized the outcomes after liver trauma over the past decades. The advents of pre-hospital care are awaited to change the need for DCS in the future.

Author details

Ioannis A. Ziogas[1†], Ioannis Katsaros[2†] and Georgios Tsoulfas[3*]

1 Division of Hepatobiliary Surgery and Liver Transplantation, Department of Surgery, Vanderbilt University Medical Center, Nashville, TN, USA

2 Department of Surgery, Metaxa Cancer Hospital, Piraeus, Greece

3 First Department of Surgery, Papageorgiou General Hospital, Aristotle University of Thessaloniki, Thessaloniki, Greece

*Address all correspondence to: tsoulfasg@gmail.com

† Both authors have contributed equally and share first co-authorship.

References

[1] David Richardson J, Franklin GA, Lukan JK, Carrillo EH, Spain DA, Miller FB, et al. Evolution in the management of hepatic trauma: a 25-year perspective. Ann Surg. 2000 Sep;232(3):324-30.

[2] Coccolini F, Montori G, Catena F, Di Saverio S, Biffl W, Moore EE, et al. Liver trauma: WSES position paper. World J Emerg Surg. 2015;10:39.

[3] Tarchouli M, Elabsi M, Njoumi N, Essarghini M, Echarrab M, Chkoff MR. Liver trauma: What current management? Hepatobiliary Pancreat Dis Int. 2018 Feb;17(1):39-44.

[4] Badger SA, Barclay R, Campbell P, Mole DJ, Diamond T. Management of liver trauma. World J Surg. 2009 Dec;33(12):2522-37.

[5] Sikhondze WL, Madiba TE, Naidoo NM, Muckart DJJ. Predictors of outcome in patients requiring surgery for liver trauma. Injury. 2007;38(1):65-70.

[6] Gao J, Du D, Zhao X, Liu G, Yang J, Zhao S, et al. Liver trauma: experience in 348 cases. World J Surg. 2003 Jun;27(6):703-8.

[7] Becker CD, Mentha G, Terrier F. Blunt abdominal trauma in adults: role of CT in the diagnosis and management of visceral injuries. Part 1: liver and spleen. Eur Radiol. 1998;8(4):553-62.

[8] Miller PR, Croce MA, Bee TK, Malhotra AK, Fabian TC. Associated injuries in blunt solid organ trauma: implications for missed injury in nonoperative management. J Trauma. 2002 Aug;53(2):234-8.

[9] Sibulesky L. Normal liver anatomy. Clin liver Dis [Internet]. 2013 Mar 29;2(Suppl 1):S1-3. Available from: https://pubmed.ncbi.nlm.nih.gov/30992874

[10] Drake R, Vogl AW, Mitchell AWM. Gray's Anatomy for Students E-Book. Elsevier Health Sciences; 2009.

[11] Couinaud C. Le foie: études anatomiques et chirurgicales. Paris: Masson; 1957.

[12] Couinaud C. Liver anatomy: portal (and suprahepatic) or biliary segmentation. Dig Surg. 1999;16(6):459-67.

[13] Skandalakis JE, Skandalakis LJ, Skandalakis PN, Mirilas P. Hepatic surgical anatomy. Surg Clin. 2004;84(2):413-35.

[14] Chen Y, Yue X, Zhong C, Wang G. Functional region annotation of liver CT image based on vascular tree. Biomed Res Int. 2016;2016.

[15] Cantlie J. On a new arrangement of the right and left lobes of the liver. J Anat Physiol. 1898;32:4-10.

[16] Smithuis R. Anatomy of the liver segments [Internet]. Radiology Assistant. 2006. Available from: https://web.archive.org/web/20150626114141/http:/www.radiologyassistant.nl/en/p4375bb8dc241d/anatomy-of-the-liver-segments.html

[17] Bismuth H. Surgical anatomy and anatomical surgery of the liver. World J Surg. 1982;6(1):3-9.

[18] Moore EE, Cogbill TH, Jurkovich GJ, Shackford SR, Malangoni MA, Champion HR. Organ injury scaling: spleen and liver (1994 revision). J Trauma Acute Care Surg. 1995;38(3):323-4.

[19] Kozar RA, Crandall M, Shanmuganathan K, Zarzaur BL,

Coburn M, Cribari C, et al. Organ injury scaling 2018 update: Spleen, liver, and kidney. J Trauma Acute Care Surg. 2018;85(6):1119-22.

[20] Coccolini F, Catena F, Moore EE, Ivatury R, Biffl W, Peitzman A, et al. WSES classification and guidelines for liver trauma. World J Emerg Surg. 2016;11(1):50.

[21] Piper GL, Peitzman AB. Current management of hepatic trauma. Surg Clin. 2010;90(4):775-85.

[22] ATLS S, group IA working. Advanced trauma life support (ATLS®): the ninth edition. J Trauma Acute Care Surg. 2013;74(5):1363.

[23] Tignanelli CJ, Joseph B, Jakubus JL, Iskander GA, Napolitano LM, Hemmila MR. Variability in management of blunt liver trauma and contribution of level of American College of Surgeons Committee on Trauma verification status on mortality. J Trauma Acute Care Surg. 2018;84(2):273-9.

[24] Scalea TM, Rodriguez A, Chiu WC, Brenneman FD, Fallon WF, Kato K, et al. Focused assessment with sonography for trauma (FAST): results from an international consensus conference. J Trauma Acute Care Surg. 1999;46(3):466-72.

[25] Yoon W, Jeong YY, Kim JK, Seo JJ, Lim HS, Shin SS, et al. CT in blunt liver trauma. Radiographics. 2005;25(1):87-104.

[26] Feliciano D V. Abdominal trauma revisited. Am Surg. 2017;83(11):1193-202.

[27] Hoff WS, Holevar M, Nagy KK, Patterson L, Young JS, Arrillaga A, et al. Practice management guidelines for the evaluation of blunt abdominal trauma: the East practice management guidelines work group. J Trauma Acute Care Surg. 2002;53(3):602-15.

[28] Edalatpour A, Young BT, Brown LR, Tseng ES, Ladhani HA, Patel NJ, et al. Grade of injury, not initial management, is associated with unplanned interventions in liver injury. Injury. 2020;

[29] Yahya AI. Damage Control in Liver Surgery. In: Tsoulfas G, editor. Surgical Challenges in the Management of Liver Disease [Internet]. Rijeka: IntechOpen; 2019. Available from: https://doi.org/10.5772/intechopen.80817

[30] Lamb CM, MacGoey P, Navarro AP, Brooks AJ. Damage control surgery in the era of damage control resuscitation. BJA Br J Anaesth [Internet]. 2014 Aug 1;113(2):242-9. Available from: https://doi.org/10.1093/bja/aeu233

[31] Pringle J. Notes on the arrest of hepatic hemorrhage due to trauma. Ann Surg. 1908;48:541-549.

[32] Halstead W. Ligature and suture material: The employment of fine silk in preference to catgut and the advantage of transfixing tissues and controlling hemorrhage—Also an account of the introduction of gloves, gutta-percha tissue and silver foil. JAMA. 1913;LX:1119-26.

[33] Leppäniemi A. Who invented damage control surgery? Scand J Surg [Internet]. 2014 Aug 5;103(3):165-6. Available from: https://doi.org/10.1177/1457496914542192

[34] Stone H, Strom P, Mullins R. Management of the major coagulopathy with onset during laparotomy. Ann Surg. 1983;197:532-5.

[35] Rotondo MF, Schwab CW, McGonigal MD, Phillips GR 3rd, Fruchterman TM, Kauder DR, et al. "Damage control": an approach for improved survival in exsanguinating penetrating abdominal injury. J Trauma. 1993 Sep;35(3):373-5.

[36] Johnson JW, Gracias VH, Schwab CW, Reilly PM, Kauder DR, Shapiro MB, et al. Evolution in damage control for exsanguinating penetrating abdominal injury. J Trauma. 2001 Aug;51(2):261-71.

[37] Dabbs DN, Stein DM, Scalea TM. Major hepatic necrosis: a common complication after angioembolization for treatment of high-grade liver injuries. J Trauma. 2009 Mar;66(3):621-9.

[38] Roberts I, Shakur H, Afolabi A, Brohi K, Coats T, Dewan Y, et al. The importance of early treatment with tranexamic acid in bleeding trauma patients: an exploratory analysis of the CRASH-2 randomised controlled trial. Lancet (London, England). 2011 Mar;377(9771):1096-101, 1101.e1-2.

[39] Hooper TJ, De Pasquale M, Strandenes G, Sunde G, Ward KR. Challenges and possibilities in forward resuscitation. Shock. 2014 May;41 Suppl 1:13-20.

[40] Holcomb JB, Jenkins D, Rhee P, Johannigman J, Mahoney P, Mehta S, et al. Damage control resuscitation: directly addressing the early coagulopathy of trauma. J Trauma. 2007 Feb;62(2):307-10.

[41] Duchesne JC, McSwain NEJ, Cotton BA, Hunt JP, Dellavolpe J, Lafaro K, et al. Damage control resuscitation: the new face of damage control. J Trauma. 2010 Oct;69(4):976-90.

[42] Schreiber MA. The beginning of the end for damage control surgery. Vol. 99 Suppl 1, The British journal of surgery. England; 2012. p. 10-1.

[43] Borgman MA, Spinella PC, Perkins JG, Grathwohl KW, Repine T, Beekley AC, et al. The ratio of blood products transfused affects mortality in patients receiving massive transfusions at a combat support hospital. J Trauma. 2007 Oct;63(4):805-13.

[44] Martinaud C, Civadier C, Ausset S, Verret C, Deshayes A-V, Sailliol A. In vitro hemostatic properties of French lyophilized plasma. Anesthesiology. 2012 Aug;117(2):339-46.

[45] Garrigue D, Godier A, Glacet A, Labreuche J, Kipnis E, Paris C, et al. French lyophilized plasma versus fresh frozen plasma for the initial management of trauma-induced coagulopathy: a randomized open-label trial. J Thromb Haemost. 2018 Mar;16(3):481-9.

[46] Jost D, Lemoine S, Lemoine F, Lanoe V, Maurin O, Derkenne C, et al. French lyophilized plasma versus normal saline for post-traumatic coagulopathy prevention and correction: PREHO-PLYO protocol for a multicenter randomized controlled clinical trial. Trials. 2020 Jan;21(1):106.

[47] Coccolini F, Coimbra R, Ordonez C, Kluger Y, Vega F, Moore EE, et al. Liver trauma: WSES 2020 guidelines. World J Emerg Surg [Internet]. 2020;15(1):24. Available from: https://doi.org/10.1186/s13017-020-00302-7

[48] Kozar RA, Feliciano D V, Moore EE, Moore FA, Cocanour CS, West MA, et al. Western Trauma Association/critical decisions in trauma: operative management of adult blunt hepatic trauma. J Trauma. 2011 Jul;71(1):1-5.

[49] Letoublon C, Reche F, Abba J, Arvieux C. Damage control laparotomy. J Visc Surg. 2011 Oct;148(5):e366-70.

[50] Letoublon C, Amariutei A, Taton N, Lacaze L, Abba J, Risse O, et al. Management of blunt hepatic trauma. J Visc Surg. 2016 Aug;153(4 Suppl):33-43.

[51] Kodadek LM, Efron DT, Haut ER. Intrahepatic Balloon Tamponade for Penetrating Liver Injury: Rarely Needed

but Highly Effective. World J Surg. 2019 Feb;43(2):486-9.

[52] Peitzman AB, Marsh JW. Advanced operative techniques in the management of complex liver injury. J Trauma Acute Care Surg. 2012 Sep;73(3):765-70.

[53] Rocca A, Andolfi E, Zamboli AGI, Surfaro G, Tafuri D, Costa G, et al. Management of complications of first instance of hepatic trauma in a liver surgery unit: Portal vein ligation as a conservative therapeutic strategy. Open Med [Internet]. 2019;14(1):376-83. Available from: https://www.degruyter.com/view/journals/med/14/1/article-p376.xml

[54] Franklin GA, Casos SR. Current advances in the surgical approach to abdominal trauma. Injury. 2006 Dec;37(12):1143-56.

[55] Mohr AM, Lavery RF, Barone A, Bahramipour P, Magnotti LJ, Osband AJ, et al. Angiographic embolization for liver injuries: low mortality, high morbidity. J Trauma. 2003 Dec;55(6):1072-7.

[56] Matsumoto S, Cantrell E, Jung K, Smith A, Coimbra R. Influence of postoperative hepatic angiography on mortality after laparotomy in Grade IV/V hepatic injuries. J Trauma Acute Care Surg. 2018 Aug;85(2):290-7.

[57] Cotton BA, Au BK, Nunez TC, Gunter OL, Robertson AM, Young PP. Predefined massive transfusion protocols are associated with a reduction in organ failure and postinjury complications. J Trauma. 2009 Jan;66(1):41-9.

Chapter 4

Liver Trauma Management

Henrique A. Wiederkehr, Julio Wiederkehr, Barbara A. Wiederkehr, Lucas M. Sarquis, Oona T. Daronch, Lucas Scopel and João V. Zeni

Abstract

Liver trauma is responsible for the majority of penetrating abdominal trauma and is the third most common injury caused by firearms. Presenting a 20% mortality rate, it is an organ with wide and complex vascularization, receiving blood from the hepatic veins and portal vein, as well as from the hepatic arteries. The diagnosis is not always simple in polytrauma patients and contains a wide range of exams such as computerized tomography and diagnostic peritoneal lavage. Treatment depends mostly on a few factors such as the patient's hemodynamic stability, the degree of injury according to the AAST classification, the resources available, and the surgeon's expertise. Considering these factors, minor lesions can be treated mostly with a conservative approach in hemodynamically stable patients. Embolization by arteriography has shown good results in major lesions in clinically stable patients as well. On the other hand, more complex lesions associated with hemodynamically unstable patients may indicate damage control surgery applying techniques such as temporary liver packing and clamping the pedicle to restore the hemodynamic status. This chapter aims to describe those techniques and their indications in liver trauma.

Keywords: liver trauma, damage control surgery, hepatic trauma, hepatic surgery, trauma surgery

1. Introduction

1.1 Liver trauma

Trauma is the leading cause of death in people aged 1–44 years, with hemorrhage being the primary cause of preventable death, accounting for 30–40% of fatalities [1]. The liver is the main organ affected in penetrating abdominal trauma in 35–45% of cases, mainly due to its susceptible and relatively superficial location in the right hypochondrium [2], and is the most commonly injured organ in patients suffering blunt abdominal trauma as well [3].

2. Incidence

Data from the National Trauma Data Bank (NTDB) showed that liver injury occurs in almost 40% of victims of blunt abdominal trauma with an overall mortality of 14.9% [4]. Liver trauma can range from minor lacerations or capsular hematomas with minimal morbidity and mortality to hepatic avulsions with high mortality.

Most hepatic injuries are minor and can be graded using the American Association for the Surgery of Trauma Hepatic Injury Scale as described under the "classification" topic ahead [5].

The right lobe of the liver, being the largest portion of the liver parenchyma, constitutes the region most affected during abdominal injury. It is known that it occurs more frequently in males and in young individuals, in the first four decades of life, in the majority of cases. Associated factors include risky behavior, such as alcohol and drug consumption, and more exposure to accidents. The mortality of patients with liver trauma ranges from 14.9–20%. When associated with shotgun lesions, the severity of the injury tends to be higher; therefore, the mortality could be up to 20% [6].

3. Classification

The severity of liver injuries is classified according to the American Association for the Surgery of Trauma (AAST) grading scale. This scale is based on parenchymal level of injury and number of liver segments affected.

To understand the classification of liver trauma, it is essential to master the anatomy of the liver. The division of the liver by the Couinaud segments occurs through the branching of the portal triad, composed of the branch of the portal vein, the hepatic artery, and the bile duct. The ramifications of these vessels cause the portal blood to be mixed with the blood in the hepatic artery in the portal spaces, which drains into the centrilobular vein, subsequently into the sublobular veins, and through the two hepatic veins, which end in the inferior vena cava. **Table 1** shows the classification of liver trauma according to the AAST.

The degree of liver injury and hemodynamic instability are important determinants in the mortality rates of patients with liver trauma as well as to determine the type of treatment to be instituted [2]. The concomitance of intra-abdominal injuries with liver trauma is common in penetrating trauma, and it is also a relevant factor

Grade of liver injury	Type of injury	Description of injury
I	Haematoma	Subcapsular, <10 % surface area
	Laceration	Capsular tear, <1 cm parenchymal depth
II	Haematoma	Subcapsular, 10–50 % surface area
		Intraparenchymal, <10 cm in diameter
	Laceration	1–3 cm parenchymal depth, <10 cm length
III	Haematoma	Subcapsular, >50 % surface area or expanding. Ruptured subcapsular or parenchymal haematoma
		Intraparenchymal haematoma >10 cm or expanding
	Laceration	>3 cm parenchymal depth
IV	Laceration	Parenchymal disruption involving 25–75 % hepatic lobe or 1-3 Couinaud's segments in a single lobe
V	Laceration	Parenchymal disruption involving >75 % of hepatic lobe or >3 Couinaud's segments within a single lobe
	Vascular	Juxtahepatic venous injuries, i.e., retrohepatic vena cava/central major hepatic veins
VI	Vascular	Hepatic avulsion

Table 1.
Classification of hepatic trauma (AAST).

in the management. [6] However, in many cases, there is no correlation between the AAST degree and the patient's physiological state [7].

Most patients have grade I injuries, and the incidence gradually decreases as the degree of injury increases, as shown by a study conducted with 300 patients between 2003 and 2013 at the Department of Surgery and Emergency, in Kartal [2]. It was found that the prognostic factors [2] related to the worst outcome were high levels of AST, ALT, LDH, INR, and creatinine and low levels of platelets and fibrinogen at admission, which were also associated with liver injuries of grades IV and V.

4. Diagnosis

Currently, the most useful complementary exams in the diagnosis of liver trauma are abdominal ultrasound and computed tomography (CT) with intravenous contrast. Abdominal ultrasound is the initial image exam, with a sensitivity of 82–88% and specificity of 99%, to detect intra-abdominal injuries, although it must be taken into account that the accuracy depends on the examiner's experience [8]. Computed tomography is the most sensitive and specific technique for determining the extent and severity of liver trauma and is the imaging test that provides us with more information on polytrauma patients, since it offers an excellent view of the skull, chest, abdomen and pelvis, bone structures, viscera, and soft tissues. The arrival of helical technology has improved the resolution, reduced the duration of the exam, and allowed the three-dimensional reconstruction of the images, which is very useful if there is vascular involvement.

Diagnosis by peritoneal lavage (LPD), with the advent of new imaging techniques, has fewer indications. Although it has an accuracy of 98% to detect intraperitoneal blood, it lacks specificity of the injured organ, which causes many unnecessary laparotomies [8].

In patients with hemodynamic instability, the Focused Assessment with Sonography for Trauma (FAST) is the exam of choice due to its sensibility to detect free fluid in the abdomen, and it can be done faster than CT as an initial exam. **Figures 1**, **2**, and **3** show some possible changes in abdominal CT in patients with liver trauma.

Some more recent studies have shown the role of two-dimensional and three-dimensional [15] ultrasonography (US) in the trauma of massive viscera, such as the liver. There is evidence that the regular US is not capable of having high

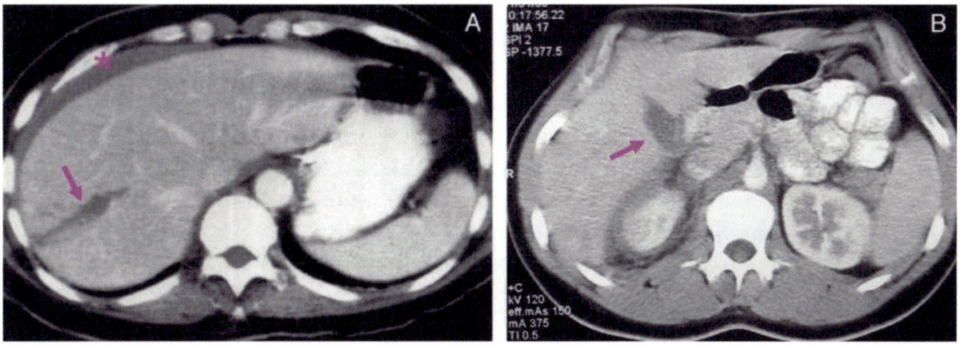

Figure 1.
Hemorrhagic hepatic lacerations (A) in the right hepatic lobe and (B) close to the hilum. Hypodense areas of linear morphology that come into contact with the capsule (arrows). They associate free liquid (asterisks).

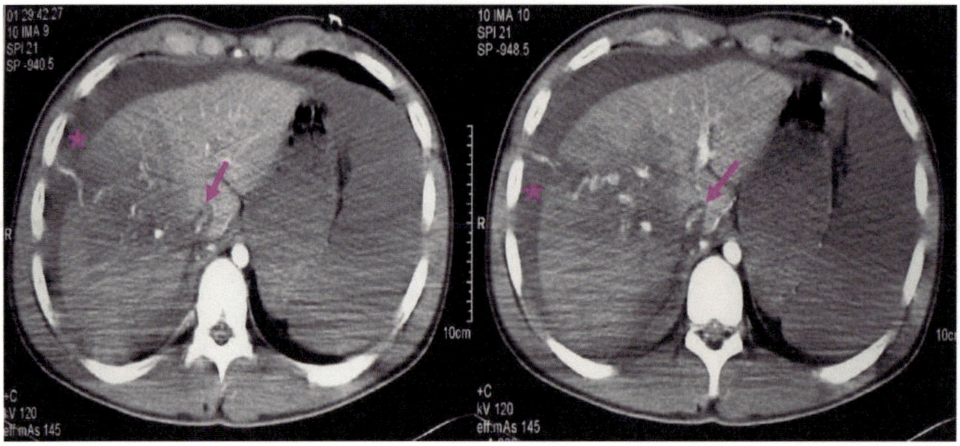

Figure 2.
Extension to the inferior vena cava. There is a large hepatic termination with extension to the inferior vena cava (arrow), which appears to be free of perihepatic primary fluid and active for bleeding (asterisk).

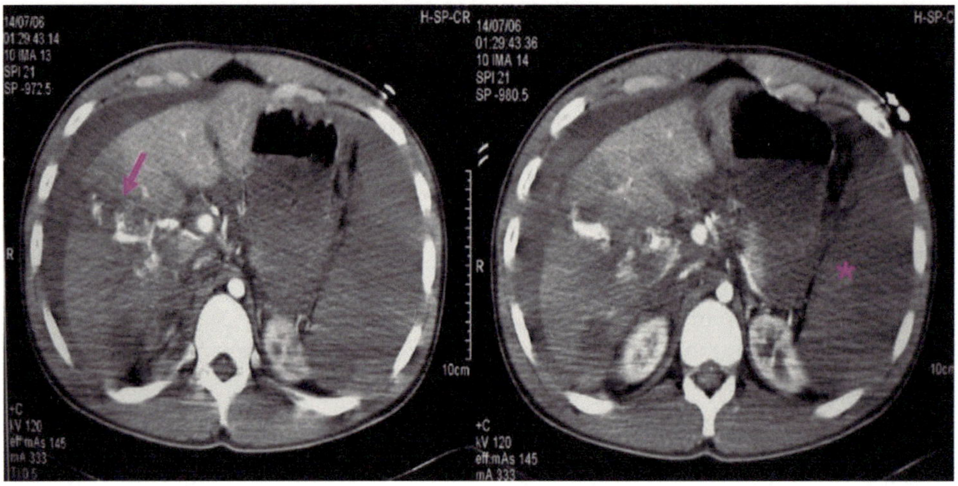

Figure 3.
Active bleeding. Active contrast leakage (arrow) is observed in a patient with severe hepatic trauma. Associated perihepatic fluid (hemoperitoneum). Splenic infarction (*).

sensitivity to detect active bleeding in a solid abdominal organ. In recent years, US using contrast agents could greatly improve the detection of bleeding. Recently, contrast US has mainly depended on two-dimensional ultrasound (2DUS). With the development of imaging technology, three-dimensional static ultrasound (3DSUS) and real-time three-dimensional ultrasound (RT3DUS) can provide more accurate images and additional information in some assessments of abdominal disease. Thus, there are new technologies and possibilities for measuring the degree of hepatic impairment, but these are not always available, and sometimes just the physical examination is possible as a diagnostic tool [8].

5. Treatment

The treatment for liver trauma has been modified over the years, since the beginning of the twentieth century, when aggressive surgical treatment predominated, which gradually changed over the decades to more conservative treatment, especially after the Second World War.

6. Indications

"Miss nothing and fix everything" has long been the dogma for emergency management of visceral trauma, which imposed obligatory emergency laparotomy for any hemoperitoneum. For blunt hepatic trauma, that attitude has been gradually transformed since the 1970s, moving toward avoidance of emergency laparotomy whenever possible [9–11]. Introduction nonoperative management of blunt liver injury has been proven to be an effective treatment option since the late 1990s, regardless of the degree of injury as long as the patient's condition remains stable [12–14].

Currently, nonoperative management is undertaken in 60–80% of blunt traumatic liver injuries, and [15, 16] the success rate is 82–100% [8, 15, 17]. The overall mortality and morbidity of those cases is 5–8 and 14–18%, respectively [15–17]. The overall mortality in surgically managed patients is 9–18%, but in high-grade injuries (grades III–V) the mortality is around 40%, and the overall morbidity in operated patients is 30–40% [15, 17]. Coimbra et al. [18] have reported that nonoperative management reduces the overall mortality of grade III and IV blunt liver injuries [19].

This approach has been supported by not only the contribution of contrast-enhanced CT [9–11] but the endoscopic and radiological adjunctive interventional procedures as well, which have expanded its scope and helped managing postoperative complications [15].

A review of the literature about the indications and effectiveness of liver angioembolization in the context of trauma showed that the main indications for this procedure are the presence of contrast blush on CT scan (the most common) and failure in nonoperative management and control of continued bleeding after damage control surgery. The authors included 11 articles related to the topic, with the rate of effectiveness of hepatic angioembolization being 93%, and the main complications highlighted were the presence of liver necrosis (15%), abscess formation (7.5%), and biliary leakage [20].

7. Surgical treatment

Despite the trend of nonoperative treatment and continued advances in the areas of trauma and critical care, uncontrolled bleeding from major liver injury is still the leading cause of death and continues to frustrate trauma surgeons [12]. Therefore, it is crucial for the surgeon to know when surgery is needed. The two most important criteria for indicating immediate operative treatment to a patient with a hepatic injury are the presence of hemodynamic instability and the existence of peritoneal irritation, regardless of the grade of injury or the volume of hemoperitoneum.

There are several surgical techniques that could be applied depending upon the complexity of the lesion including simple manual compression, Pringle's maneuver (clamping of the hepatoduodenal ligament), hepatorrhaphy, hepatectomy, hepatic artery ligation, and liver resection. Finally, in the direst of circumstances and under specific indications, even a liver transplant can be considered [6]. Regarding the incidence of the surgical techniques employed, hepatorrhaphy is generally the most used procedure in most cases, and the least used are epiplonplasty and left hepatectomy, according to a recently published study, as shown in **Table 2** [6].

Technique*	Patients	%
Hepatorrhaphy	86	80.37
Segmentectomy	2	1.87
Left hepatectomy	1	0.93
Electrocauterization	4	3.74
Topical hemostatic agents	2	1.87
Epiploplasty	1	0.93
Damage Control	7	6.54
No action (liver damage with no active bleeding)	12	11.21
Nontherapeutic laparotomy	4	3.74

Table 2.
Surgical techniques used to treat liver injuries in patients with liver trauma.

8. Damage control surgery

8.1 Background

Besides all advances portrayed, the prognosis of hemodynamically unstable patients with complex (AAST Organ Injury Scale 4 IV–V) liver injury is still poor, as their treatment and decision-making process are extremely challenging for the trauma team [21]. It is known that approximately 10% of the patients in this scenario will present life-threatening injuries and hemodynamic shock and that the primary and ultimate repair of severe traumatic injuries in patients with unstable physiology is detrimental to outcome [1, 22, 23]. A staged management approach known as "damage control surgery" (DCS) has been demonstrated to improve the survival in these cases [1, 22]. The principles of DCS involve abbreviated surgery to control blood loss and contamination in the abdomen with simultaneous resuscitation of physiology. Once the hemodynamic state is restored, the definitive surgical repair is performed [22, 24].

Although the term "damage control surgery" was first described for trauma management by Rotondo et al. [22], the idea of the procedure was already existent for a long time before. The proposal to use this surgery in trauma and emergencies has succeed during the Second World War, in the mid-1940s, when the structure for hospital care was insufficient and the number of victims exceeded the capacity to give support to the injured [25]. There are older reports of the application of this technique with similar purposes in Edwin Smith's Surgical Papyrus, more than 8000 years ago, a conduct used by the absence of other options at the time the idea was conceived [26].

According to a review by Benz and Balogh about damage control surgery, its modern model emerged in the late 1970s from clinical experience with major hepatic trauma [27]. Perihepatic packing consists in manually approximating the liver parenchyma followed by the consecutive placing of dry abdominal packs around the liver and straight over the injury. This technique was firstly incorporated by Pringle [28] in enthusiasm for staged laparotomy. Since then, numerous clinical reviews were conducted in order to study this technique.

Elerding et al. [29] observed that 82% of deaths following liver trauma were due to uncontrolled hemorrhage and progressive coagulopathy, even after primary vascular injuries had been addressed. The whole lethal coagulopathic state apparently was impaired by hypothermia and acidosis, the observation upon which the "lethal triad" term was suggested [23]. In 1981, Feliciano et al. [30] reported on the observed merit of temporary laparotomy pad tamponade for postinjury coagulopathy. Nine out of 10 patients with persistent hepatic parenchymal ooze, despite all attempts at surgical control, survived with intra-abdominal packing and delayed removal. This finding led the authors to advocate the technique as a lifesaving maneuver in select trauma patients with persistent coagulopathy. Two years later, Svoboda et al. [31] reaffirmed the survival benefit of intra-abdominal packing.

Despite being initially organized as an emergency strategy in patients who have suffered severe trauma, the principles of damage control have also been approached in nontraumatic abdominal emergencies, in order to reduce mortality compared to definitive primary surgery [32]. According to the 10th edition of ATLS [33], damage control surgery is an important component of crisis management care, given that in many disasters, hospitals are destroyed and transportation to medical facilities may not be feasible or the environment may be contaminated, so this context is an option for using this technique.

8.2 Intra-abdominal packing

Damage control surgery by intra-abdominal packing has shown to be effective and able to significantly decrease morbidity and mortality, both in trauma and nontraumatic massive intra-abdominal hemorrhage [34]. In the last decades, consensus has been reached about considering the accomplishment of an effective perihepatic packing [35] to be the most effective and quickest way in order to obtain hemorrhage control [21].

This procedure consists in the placement, after fast and complete mobilization of the right liver lobe, of a total number of eight lap pads all around the posterior paracaval surface (avoiding vena cava compression), the lateral right side, the anterior surface, and posteroinferior visceral surface of the liver (avoiding any intrahepatic packing) [36, 45]. The diaphragmatic surface must remain free in order to avoid any respiratory compromise. Reoperation after appropriate resuscitation allows packing removal and definitive repair of liver injuries.

8.3 Indications for damage control surgery

Regarding the indications for damage control surgery, it is known that there is a wide range of conditions in which it can be used, and the decisive moment for the use of these techniques is not preoperative adequacy, but the intraoperative becomes essential for the evaluation [37].

Overall, in the context of severe trauma with hemodynamic instability, the rationale of performing a "shortened laparotomy" is usually based upon the concept of the lethal triad [25], composed of hypothermia (due to inadequate environmental conditions, deficient thermal protection, blood loss, and infusion of unheated liquids), metabolic acidosis (inadequate tissue perfusion, caused by hemorrhage and shock, which predisposes to anaerobic metabolism and metabolic acidosis), and coagulopathy (metabolic acidosis with interference on coagulation factors and volume replacement).

In a practical manner, there are some absolute indications for the procedure, such as estimated blood loss greater than 4 L and the administration of more than 10 red blood cell concentrates [37]. Although there are classic indications for performing damage control surgery, new studies have questioned these indications and proposed other observations to better elucidate the cases eligible for the procedure [37]. Among them, those who presented moderate accuracy were systolic blood pressure (BP) < 90 mmHg or central body temperature < 34°C, and five indications produced major and conclusive changes in the pretest probability of performing damage control surgery during emerging laparotomy: discovery of pancreas, duodenum, or pancreatic-duodenal complex devascularized or completely ruptured;

a. Large abdominal vascular lesions with multiple visceral lesions
b. Diffuse bleeding of a nonmechanical nature
c. Multiple trunk penetrations
d. Blunt trunk trauma, resulting from high-energy impact
e. Operating and resuscitation time greater than 90 minutes
f. Bulky transfusion (>10 red blood cell concentrates)
g. Severe liver damage
h. Ruptured pelvic hematomas
i. Lesions of the retrohepatic vena cava
j. Pancreatic lesions that require resection
k. Significant hemodynamic instability

Table 3.
Traditional indications of damage control surgery.

estimated intraoperative blood loss >4 L; administration of >10 U of concentrate and red blood cells; and systolic BP persistently <90 mmHg or arterial pH persistently <7.2 during the operation [37]. The traditional indications [38] to perform this surgery are explained in **Table 3**. The factors related to almost 100% of mortality [25] are temperature (value <32°C), advanced age (70 years), and drop in pH.

Damage control surgery can be performed in three basic and sequential steps [25], which consist of the following:

a. Performing lifesaving procedures, such as stopping bleeding, controlling evisceration, and avoiding resections and reconstructions.

b. Resuscitation in an intensive care unit (ICU).

c. New surgical approach intended to review the lesions and to attempt definitive treatment.

Although it is often the only option in severe trauma, surgery to control damage should be considered, since it is related to serious complications [39], such as enteric fistulas, readmissions, multiple surgical interventions, and reduced quality of life.

In a study carried out in a trauma center in the city of Sao Paulo, Brazil, from a total of 392 patients, 207 had liver damage, and in cases it was necessary to perform the DCS (6.54%), which showed 100% survival, reaffirming the role of damage control surgery in severely traumatized patients with the lethal triad [6].

9. Liver transplantation in hepatic trauma

Considering that the causes of death following severe hepatic trauma are uncontrollable bleeding due to vascular and liver laceration injury and acute liver failure, it is possible to cogitate liver transplantation as an option, since the procedure could treat both conditions; however, indications are still very restricted [40–42].

The indications for liver transplantation in this scenario described in the literature are uncontrollable continuous bleeding after damage control operation; extensive complex liver lacerations not amenable to surgical correction; extensive lesions of the portal vein, hepatic vein, or bile duct that cannot be repaired by surgery; progressive liver failure due to trauma; and hepatic necrosis [40–42].

It is important to keep in mind that this procedure should only be considered once all other therapies were attempted, making it imperative to adopt damage control measures in order to promote temporary hemostasis until an organ becomes available for transplantation [38–41]. Also, not all patients are candidates for transplant and that the choice should be conducted carefully and individually. Situations such as severe sepsis, multiple organ failure, and other associated serious injuries may contraindicate the transplant [40–43].

There are two types of procedures described in the literature: transplantation in one step and staged transplantation. The first consists in the immediate removal of the native liver with subsequent implantation of a new organ, whereas the latter consists in creating a temporary vascular portocaval shunt to allow the patient to wait for the organ and avoid congestion in mesenteric splanchnic system [40, 42].

It is important to keep in mind that this is the last alternative to serious hepatic lesions. Even when indicated, this treatment presents a low success rate not being a viable alternative to the majority of liver traumas.

10. Complications

Trauma patients, especially those requiring a staged surgical approach, are subjected to multiple operations and prolonged ICU stays and are at high risk of developing complications such as abdominal compartment syndrome (ACS), acute respiratory distress syndrome, and multiple organ failure.

Generally, the incidence of complications is related to the degree of the hepatic trauma and the type of treatment used in the process, being directly proportional to the severity of the trauma presented by the patient, ranging from small changes in the liver parenchyma to vascular and biliary system injuries.

Since the majority of the liver injuries are managed nonoperatively, it is important to bear in mind that approximately a quarter of the patients with blunt hepatic injury managed nonoperatively will manifest complications that impose intervention, infrequently operative [3].

There is evidence that conservative treatment for extensive liver injuries results in a higher incidence of biliovascular complications [44]. In a recent article carried out in Italy with 56 young patients with liver injury AAST III or greater, mostly due to blunt trauma, 17 patients had 21 liver complications: 4 biliary, 12 vascular, and 1 combined biliary and vascular. Liver complications increased with the highest degree of liver trauma, with 3.5% in grade III, 52% in grade IV, and 70% in grade V. One patient with active arterio-portal fistula required urgent angioembolization, while other arterial pseudoaneurysms 7.23 ± 5.14 days after the trauma were detected. Angioembolization was successful in 83% of patients. The work highlighted that the main predictors of biliovascular complications were the requirement for blood transfusion and the degree of injury. Portal vein laceration was a predictor of biliary and nonvascular complications [44].

When considering radiological intervention, as portrayed previously, the main complication of hepatic angioembolization is the presence of massive hepatic necrosis (MHN). In a study carried out with 538 patients who had high-grade traumatic liver injuries [6], 16 patients (22.5%) had grade III injuries, 44 (62%) grade IV injuries, and 11 (15.5%) grade V injuries, with 71 (13%) having undergone therapeutic liver angioembolization, with 8 patients (11.3%) from the latter group dying as a result of liver damage. Complication rates were 18.8%, 65.9%, and 100% in patients with grade III, IV, and V injuries, respectively, for an overall complication rate of

60.6%. Thirty patients (42.2%) developed MHN [45]. Patients who developed MHN were compared with those who did not. It was observed that patients with MHN had higher-grade lesions, significantly needed more transfusions, and had a significantly longer hospital stay (all $p < 0.001$). Patients who developed MHN were more likely to undergo surgical intervention (96.7% vs. 41.5%, $p < 0.001$), with 87% undergoing damage control laparotomy [45].

As for the surgical treatment, many complications can occur depending on the type of procedure. The most frequent postoperative complication is related to infection such as pneumonia, peritonitis, and intra-abdominal abscess, and it represents almost three quarters of all immediate complications. The survival rate in patients with blunt liver trauma (60%) may be lower than the ones with penetrating trauma (87.5%), possibly due to the higher rate of head injuries associated with blunt trauma, as a consequence of severe traumatic brain injury [6].

In a recent study [6] carried out in a university hospital, in Sao Paulo, from 392 trauma patients who underwent laparotomy, 107 had liver injuries, 78.5% with penetrating trauma, in severe firearm injuries. The incidence of postoperative complications was 29.9%, and the most frequent were infections, including pneumonia, peritonitis, and intra-abdominal abscess. The survival rate of patients with blunt trauma was 60% and of penetrating trauma, 87.5% ($p < 0.05$). Another retrospective work carried out at the Department of Hepatobiliary Surgery and Liver Transplantation Unit of A.O.R.N.A. Cardarelli from Naples, Italy, considered 50 patients with liver trauma and assessed the main complications related to the type of trauma and treatment employed [46]. A wide range of complications is observed and is associated with five pathophysiological findings: acute bleeding after packing the cavity with compresses, liver hematoma, arteriovenous fistula, sepsis, biliary fistula, and coleperitoneum [46].

With the implementation of DCS, patients previously considered as beyond help turned capable of surviving their initial injuries, and as they were transferred to ICUs for physiological stabilization prior to surgical reconstruction, they were submitted through a supranormal resuscitation [1]. Later it was observed that this practice resulted in many of these patients receiving excessive volumes of crystalloid and experiencing subsequent problematic tissue edema of the lungs and gut during attempts at physiological restoration [47]. The combination of shock, large volume resuscitation, intestinal edema, and a tightly packed and closed abdomen led to increased intra-abdominal pressures and the development of virtual epidemics of abdominal compartment syndrome [47]. With an initial reported prevalence of more than 30% and mortality rate greater than 60% [48] in the major trauma population, many patients died not from their initial injuries but from lethal respiratory, renal, and cardiac failure due to increased abdominal pressure. Prospective observational studies soon identified the association between abdominal compartment syndrome and traumatic shock resuscitation [1, 49].

The aggravated physiologic derangement caused by intra-abdominal hypertension (IAH) can rapidly result in multiorgan failure in a vicious circle unless interrupted by abdominal decompression [50–52] such as open abdomen management (OA). OA consists of intentionally leaving the abdominal fascial edges of the paired rectus abdominis muscles unapproximated (laparostomy) in order to abbreviate operation, prevent IAH, and facilitate reexploration without damaging the abdominal fascia. Temporary abdominal closure (TAC) refers to the method for providing protection to the abdominal viscera during the time the fascia remains open [50, 52] Patients undergoing OA management are at risk of developing entero-atmospheric fistula (EAF) and a "frozen abdomen," intra-abdominal abscesses, and lower rates of definitive fascial closure [53, 54]. The risk-benefit ratio must be kept in mind, and measures to mitigate complications are necessary. In all patients with an OA, every effort should be exerted to achieve primary fascial closure (i.e., fascia-to-fascia closure of the abdominal wall within the index hospitalization) as soon as the patient can physiologically tolerate it [50].

Through the liberal use of open abdomen surgery and systematic evidence-based modifications to traumatic shock resuscitation techniques, the concept of damage control resuscitation was created. Damage control resuscitation differs from previous resuscitation approaches by attempting an earlier and more aggressive correction of coagulopathy as well as metabolic derangements. It embraces several key concepts, including permissive hypotension, the restriction of isotonic fluid for plasma volume expansion, and the early and rapid administration of component transfusion therapy to support correction of postinjury coagulopathy [1, 55]. Damage control resuscitation restores physiological reserve facilitating more definitive surgical treatment resulting in decreased perioperative complications and improved outcomes [1].

Liver injury management has been changed in recent years with the advancement of technology, newer diagnosis, and therapeutic tools. The indications of nonoperative treatment are increasing with improvement of survival and lower morbidity rates.

11. Conclusion

The liver is the second most common affected organ in abdominal trauma and therefore has a prominent role in all the abdominal traumas. During the past decade, the management presented a significant evolution especially with the growth of interventional radiology. Procedures such as arteriography and arterial embolization helped to manage once difficult lesions with poor prognosis. Nevertheless, when it is possible, the nonoperative management should be preferred since it presents less morbidity.

Hepatic lesions classified as grade IV are a cause for anguish and anxiety for the surgeons, since they present a higher morbidity and mortality. The first concern in severe liver trauma should be the patient stabilization, which can be done through damage control surgery, which consists of executing the crucial and strategically ordered steps (shortened surgery, correction of physiological measurements in intensive care and proposed reoperation) to reduce operational time, correct a loss of death (medicated by acidosis, hypothermia, and coagulopathy), and improve the patient's long-term prognosis.

In the context of trauma, control damage surgery appears as an alternative for severely injured patients, who have multiple injuries to the abdominal viscera.

After clinical stabilization in an intensive care unit, the patient will be reoperated, and less severe injuries will be corrected, with the patient's gradual recovery after correcting the lethal triad.

In the same perspective, this chapter reviewed liver trauma centered on damage control surgery, providing the main content related to the topic, from its causes, trauma mechanism, classification, bibliographic review, therapeutic options, and current statistics to prognosis and the role of damage control surgery in this context. Thus, it is expected that at the end of the chapter, the reader will be able to organize the main topics related to liver trauma and consider making difficult decisions in practice in trauma hospital, always seeking the best prognosis for patients.

Author details

Henrique A. Wiederkehr[1], Julio Wiederkehr[2*], Barbara A. Wiederkehr[3], Lucas M. Sarquis[4], Oona T. Daronch[1], Lucas Scopel[1] and João V. Zeni[1]

1 Clinical Hospital, Federal University of Paraná, Curitiba, Paraná, Brazil

2 Federal University of Paraná, Curitiba, Paraná, Brazil

3 Vita Hospital, Curitiba, Paraná, Brazil

4 Mackenzie University Hospital, Curitiba, Paraná, Brazil

*Address all correspondence to: julio.wieder@gmail.com

References

[1] Benz D, Balogh ZJ. Damage control surgery: Current state and future directions. Current Opinion in Critical Care. 2017;**23**(6):491-497. DOI: 10.1097/MCC.0000000000000465

[2] Kaptanoglu L, Kurt N, Sikar HE. Current approach to liver traumas. International Journal of Surgery. 2017;**39**:255-259

[3] Ward J, Alarcon L, Peitzman AB. Management of blunt liver injury: What is new? European Journal of Trauma and Emergency Surgery. 2015;**41**(3):229-237. DOI: 10.1007/s00068-015-0521-0

[4] NTDB Annual Report 2017. [Accessed: 12 January 2018]

[5] Ahmed I, Beckingham IJ. Liver trauma. Trauma. 2007;**9**(3):171-180. DOI: 10.1177/1460408607086775

[6] Kalil M, Amaral IMA. Avaliação epidemiológica de vítimas de trauma hepático submetidas a tratamento cirúrgico. Revista do Colégio Brasileiro de Cirurgiões. 2016;**43**(1):22-27

[7] Coccolini F, Catena F, Moore E, Ivatury R, Biffl W, Peitzman W, et al. WSES classification and guidelines for liver trauma. World Journal of Emergency Surgery: WJES. 2016;**11**:50

[8] Sánchez-Bueno F, Fernández-Carrión J, Torres Salmerón G, García Pérez R, Ramírez Romero P, Fuster Quiñonero M, et al. Cambios en el manejo diagnóstico-terapéutico del traumatismo hepático. Estudio retrospectivo comparando 2 series de casos en periodos diferentes (1997-1984 vs. 2001-2008). Cirugía Española. 2011;**89**(7):439-447

[9] Letoublon C, Amariutei A, Taton N, Lacaze L, Abba J, Risse O, et al. Management of blunt hepatic trauma. Journal of Visceral Surgery. 2016;**153**(4):33-43. DOI: 10.1016/j.jviscsurg.2016.07.005

[10] Richardson JD. Changes in the management of injuries to the liver and spleen. Journal of the American College of Surgeons. 2005;**200**:648-669

[11] Letoublon C, Abba J, Arvieux C. Traumatismes fermes du foie. Principes de tactique et de technique chirurgicales. EMC Techniques chirurgicales-Appareil Digestif. 2012:1-23 [Article 40-785]

[12] Lin BC, Fang JF, Chen RJ, Wong YC, Hsu YP. Surgical management and outcome of blunt major liver injuries: Experience of damage control laparotomy with perihepatic packing in one trauma Centre. Injury. 2014;**45**(1):122-127. DOI: 10.1016/j.injury.2013.08.022

[13] Carrillo EH, Platz A, Miller FB, Richardson JD, Polk JC Jr. Non-operative management of blunt hepatic trauma. The British Journal of Surgery. 1998;**85**:461-468

[14] Knudson MM, Maull KI. Nonoperative management of solid organ injuries: Past, present, and future. The Surgical Clinics of North America. 1999;**79**:1357-1371

[15] Srinivasan T, Wig JD, Gupta R, Yadav TD, Doley RP, Kudari A, et al. Complex hepatic injuries: An audit from a tertiary center. European Journal of Trauma and Emergency Surgery. 2008;**34**(3):287-293. DOI: 10.1007/s00068-007-7058-9

[16] Kozar RA, Moore FA, Cothren CC, Moore EE, Sena M, Bulger EM, et al. Risk factors for hepatic morbidity following nonoperative management: Multicenter study. Archives of Surgery. 2006;**141**:451-459

[17] Christmas AB, Wilson AK, Manning B, Franklin GA, Miller FB,

Richardson JD, et al. Selective management of blunt hepatic injuries including nonoperative management is a safe and effective strategy. Surgery. 2005;**138**:606-610

[18] Coimbra R, Hoyt DB, Engelhart S, Fortlage D. Nonoperative management reduces the overall mortality of grades 3 and 4 blunt liver injuries. International Surgery. 2006;**91**:251-257

[19] Trunkey DD. Hepatic trauma: Contemporary management. The Surgical Clinics of North America. 2004;**84**:437-450

[20] Green CS, Bulger EM, Kwan SW. Outcomes and complications of angioembolization for hepatic trauma: A systematic review of the literature. Journal of Trauma and Acute Care Surgery. 2016;**80**(3):529-537

[21] DiSaverio S, Sibilio A, et al. A proposed algorithm for multimodal liver trauma management from a surgical trauma audit in a western European trauma center. Minerva Anestesiologica. 2014;**80**(11):1205-1216. Available from: http://www.embase.com/search/results?subaction=viewrecord&from=export&id=L604424378

[22] Rotondo MF, Schwab CW, McGonigal MD, et al. 'Damage control': An approach for improved survival in exsanguinating penetrating abdominal injury. The Journal of Trauma. 1993;**35**:375-382

[23] Moore EE. Thomas G. Orr Memorial Lecture. Staged laparotomy for the hypothermia, acidosis, and coagulopathy syndrome. American Journal of Surgery. 1996;**172**:405-410

[24] Rotondo MF, Zonies DH. The damage control sequence and underlying logic. The Surgical Clinics of North America. 1997;**77**:761-777

[25] Neves BHA, Mata CSR, Vaz GV, Pereira JIB, Pereira KD, Vasconcelos NM, et al. Cirurgia para controle de danos: revisão. Revista Medica de Minas Gerais. 2012;**22** (Supl 5):S14-S17

[26] Lima RAC, Macêdo PR. Cirurgia para controle do dano: Uma revisão. Revista do Colégio Brasileiro de Cirurgiões. 2007;**34**(4):257-263

[27] Walt AJ. Founder's lecture: The mythology of hepatic trauma: Or babel revisited. American Journal of Surgery. 1978;**135**:12-18

[28] Pringle JHV. Notes on the arrest of hepatic hemorrhage due to trauma. Annals of Surgery. 1908;**48**:541-549

[29] Elerding SC, Aragon GE, Moore EE. Fatal hepatic hemorrhage after trauma. American Journal of Surgery. 1979;**138**:883-888

[30] Feliciano DV, Mattox KL, Jordan GL Jr. Intra-abdominal packing for control of hepatic hemorrhage: A reappraisal. The Journal of Trauma. 1981;**21**:285-290

[31] Svoboda JA, Peter ET, Dang CV, et al. Severe liver trauma in the face of coagulopathy. A case for temporary packing and early reexploration. American Journal of Surgery. 1982;**144**:717-721

[32] Weber DG, Bendinelli C, Balogh ZJ. Damage control surgery for abdominal emergencies. The British Journal of Surgery. 2014;**101**(1):e109-e118. DOI: 10.1002/bjs.9360. Epub 2013 Nov 25

[33] American College of Surgeons; Advanced Trauma Life Support (ATLS). 10th ed, 2018

[34] Filicori F, Di Saverio S, Casali M, Biscardi A, Baldoni F, Tugnoli G. Packing for damage control of nontraumatic intra-abdominal massive hemorrhages. World Journal of Surgery. 2010;**34**:2064-2068

[35] Caruso DM, Battistella FD, Owings JT, Lee SL, Samaco RC. Perihepatic packing of major liver injuries: complications and mortality. Archives of Surgery. 1999;**134**:958-962; discusion 962-963

[36] Tarchouli M et al. Hepatobiliary & Pancreatic Diseases International. 2018. PMID: 29428102

[37] Roberts DJ, Stelfox HT, Moore LJ, Cotton BA, Holcomb JB, Harvin JA. Accuracy of published indications for predicting use of damage control during laparotomy for trauma. Journal of Surgical Research. 2019;**248**:45-55

[38] Eldemuth RCL, Buscariolli YS, Junior MAFR. Cirurgia para controle de danos: Estado atual. Revista do Colégio Brasileiro de Cirurgiões. 2013;**40**(2):142-151

[39] Pimente SK, Rucinski T, de Araújo Meskau MP, Cavassin GP, Kohl NH. Damage control surgery: Are we losing control over indications? Revista do Colégio Brasileiro de Cirurgiões. 2018;**45**(1):e1474

[40] Ribeiro-Jr MAF, Medrado MB, Rosa OM, de Deus Silva AJ, Fontana MP, Cruvinel-Neto J, et al. Liver transplantation after severe hepatic trauma: Current indications and results. Arquivos Brasileiros de Cirurgia Digestiva: ABCD = Brazilian Archives of Digestive Surgery. 2015;**28**(4):286-289. DOI: 10.1590/S0102-6720201500040017

[41] Heuer M, Kaiser GM, Lendemans S, Vernadakis S, Treckmann JW, Paul A. Transplantation after blunt trauma to the liver: A valuable option or just "waste of organs"? European Journal of Medical Research. 2010;**15**:169-173

[42] Delis SG, Bakoyiannis A, Selvaggi G, Weppler D, Levi D, Tzakis AG. Liver transplantation for severe hepatic trauma: Experience from a single center. World Journal of Gastroenterology. 2009;**15**(13):1641-1644

[43] Tucker ON, Marriott P, Mohamed R, Heaton N. Emergency liver transplantation following severe liver trauma. Liver Transplantation. 2008;**14**:1204-1210

[44] Sakaray YR, Gupta V, Yadav TD, Kalra N, Singh V. Biliovascular complications: A price to pay for non-operative management of major liver trauma. Minerva Chirurgica. 2019;**74**(5):385-391

[45] Dabbs DN, Stein DM, Scalea TM. Major hepatic necrosis: A common complication after angioembolization for treatment of high-grade liver injuries. Minerva Chirurgica. 2019;**74**(5):385-391

[46] Rocca A, Andolfi E, Zamboli AGI, Surfaro G, Tafuri D, Costa G, et al. Management of complications of first instance of hepatic trauma in a liver surgery unit: Portal vein ligation as a conservative therapeutic strategy. Open Medicine (Wars). 2019;**14**:376-383

[47] Balogh Z, McKinley BA, Cocanour CS, et al. Supranormal trauma resuscitation causes more cases of abdominal compartment syndrome. Archives of Surgery. 2003;**138**:637-642

[48] Ivatury RR, Porter JM, Simon RJ, et al. Intra-abdominal hypertension after life- threatening penetrating abdominal trauma: Prophylaxis, incidence, and clinical relevance to gastric mucosal pH and abdominal compartment syndrome. The Journal of Trauma. 1998;**44**:1016-1021

[49] Balogh ZJ, Martin A, van Wessem KP, et al. Mission to eliminate postinjury abdominal compartment syndrome. Archives of Surgery. 2011;**146**:938-943

[50] Coccolini F, Roberts D, Ansaloni L, Ivatury R, Gamberini E, Kluger Y, et al. The open abdomen in trauma and non-trauma patients: WSES guidelines. World Journal of Emergency Surgery. 2018;**13**(1):1-16. DOI: 10.1186/s13017-018-0167-4

[51] Bailey J, Shapiro MJ. Abdominal compartment syndrome. Critical Care. 2000;**4**:23-29

[52] Sartelli M, Abu-Zidan FM, Ansaloni L, Bala M, Beltrán MA, Biffl WL, et al. The role of the open abdomen procedure in managing severe abdominal sepsis: WSES position paper. World Journal of Emergency Surgery : WJES. 2015;**10**:35

[53] Coccolini F, Biffl W, Catena F, Ceresoli M, Chiara O, Cimbanassi S, et al. The open abdomen, indications, management and definitive closure. World Journal of Emergency Surgery: WJES. 2015;**10**:32

[54] Sartelli M, Catena F, Ansaloni L, Coccolini F, Corbella D, Moore EE, et al. Complicated intra-abdominal infections worldwide: The definitive data of the CIAOW study. World Journal of Emergency Surgery: WJES. 2014;**9**:37

[55] Holcomb JB, Jenkins D, Rhee P, et al. Damage control resuscitation: Directly addressing the early coagulopathy of trauma. The Journal of Trauma. 2007;**62**:307-310

Section 3

Damage Control Surgery in Different Surgical Specialties

Chapter 5

Damage Control in Hinchey III and IV Acute Diverticulitis

Luca Ponchietti, Néstor Bueno Vidales, Andrea A. Casamassima, Fernando Gallego Estrada, Alessandro Garcea, Ioannis Gerogiannis, Alberto Lafita López, Diego Mariani, Olga Marin Casajús, Matteo Marconi, Nuno Filipe Muralha Antunes, Laura María Pradal Jarne, Jorge Vera Bella and Carlos Yánez Benítez

Abstract

Acute diverticulitis is one of the most common surgical causes of admission to Emergency Departments in Western Countries. Although most of the cases can be managed conservatively or electively, a number of them will require an emergency surgical treatment. Among these patients, an even smaller number of them will present with a full-blown catastrophic septic shock. These minorities of cases have accounted for a significant part of the overall mortality and morbidity of complicated acute diverticulitis itself. The implementation of Damage Control strategies has shown to be useful also in these septic catastrophes, where a profound derangement of physiology makes unsafe a classic approach. Damage Control, as we intend it, is not a surgical "technique." A close collaboration between different specialties brought forth a strategy of treatment. The Surgeon, the Anesthetist, and the Intensivist are the three most involved specialists in the treatment of these cases. It is paramount for them to learn how to work side by side and in harmony, since the patients will benefit from each-one's input in their care.

Keywords: acute diverticulitis, damage control, peritonitis, laparostomy, Sepsis

1. Introduction

Diverticular disease is a common and increasing cause of emergency consultation in Western countries with 3–5 cases per 100,000 habitants. Although in most cases it remains asymptomatic, roughly 20% may require emergency treatment. The advances both in image quality of new multi-slice CT scans and laparoscopic procedures have influenced changes in the way we treat these complicated patients. Complications of sigmoid diverticulitis due to acute inflammation and colonic wall perforation may manifest as pericolic (Hinchey I) or extra-mesocolic (Hinchey II) abscesses, and purulent (Hinchey III) or fecal peritonitis (Hinchey IV). Although the first two are managed conservatively, treatment for stages III/IV is not that straightforward. We will refer to Hinchey III/IV acute diverticulitis as complicated acute diverticulitis (CAD) [1–3].

The clinical and surgical approach to CAD differs basically on the physiological status of the presenting patient [4].

Fortunately enough, even if CAD is, by definition, severe sepsis, a good proportion of the patients are not in septic shock at presentation. This means that they are still in a physiological state to tolerate a definitive "classical" procedure. Standard surgical therapy for CAD has been to perform either an open or laparoscopic resection, followed by a primary anastomosis or a protected anastomosis or a terminal colostomy. The latter is still the most common procedure. In recent years, a less invasive approach has been used to fit patients with Hinchey III peritonitis. In these cases, a laparoscopic lavage and drainage (LLD) seem to be, according to a growing number of surgeons, a safe option [1–6].

In this chapter, we will not linger any longer on these previous strategies.

We will focus only on the smaller group of patients with CAD who present with such an advanced derangement of their physiology that needs to be treated in a Damage Control Modality.

Damage Control, in our view, is not merely a surgical technique. It is in fact, a strategy of treatment brought forward by a close collaboration between different specialties, among which surgery, intensive care (ICU) and anesthesia play a significant role. Thus, we will present the input on each of these specialties on the therapeutic strategy.

2. Assessing the patient

We can think, out-of-the-book, abdominal emergencies as a devilish blend of dangerous ingredients. Diagnosing an acute abdomen is sorting out the different components from the mix to finally draw conclusions on its danger.

Ideally, we should be able to do it quickly, pragmatically, and in a cost-effective manner.

We appreciate that there is a significant disparity in what can be used in different health systems. What is readily available in high-income countries, it is not (or is inexistent) in low-income countries. The authors' bias is to work in some of the best health systems in the world, at least according to the World Health Organization, where almost everything is available 24/7/365.

We all know the signs and symptoms of a patient with acute diverticulitis.

They usually have persistent moderate to severe abdominal pain with guarding and rebound tenderness located in the left lower quadrant or hypogastrium (Hinchey I–II), which turns to be diffused to all the abdominal cavity as the infection is no longer localized (Hinchey III–IV).

Nausea, vomiting, fever, and in some cases, dysuria can also be present in many patients.

In modern and mature health care systems, patients with diffuse peritonitis and septic shock should be diagnosed straightforwardly with a CT abdomen-pelvis with intravenous contrast. We never stress enough to our trainees, and during our M&M, how a speedy diagnosis contributes to saving lives. Also, we are very adamant that a CT without IV contrast is a suboptimal examination in almost all the emergency clinical situations. Acute kidney injury (AKI) or chronic renal failure (CRF) are not, and should not be a contraindication to obtain a good quality CT scan. The quantity of literature on the safety of modern IV contrasts is vast and easily searchable in PubMed.

CT scan gives us all the information we need; such as free fluid vs. localized collection, the distribution of free air, and direct signs of diverticulitis. Not infrequently, it informs us of other unknown conditions that could change the overall attitude such as multiple liver metastases, primary neoplasms of the large bowel or other organs, etc.

We agree that diagnosis is paramount, but treatment is our real goal. And treatment should start before diagnosis.

An acute abdomen is a diagnosis based on clinical examination. Sepsis should be considered as the primary cause of an acute abdomen until proven otherwise. Sepsis can be identified within minutes by recognizing hypotension, tachycardia, tachypnea, and oliguria. Blood tests (White Blood Cells and C-Reactive Protein) together with venous or arterial blood gases (lactates) can add crucial information towards the final diagnosis of sepsis. Are they septic? Are they in septic shock? Usually, in acute diffuse peritonitis, from diverticulitis or other causes as well, the answer is many times, yes, they are already in septic shock. Some Health Systems, like the United Kingdom's National Health System (NHS), introduced the "Sepsis-Six." The Sepsis-Six consists of three diagnostic and three therapeutic steps—all to be delivered within 1 h of the initial diagnosis of sepsis [7]:

1. Titrate oxygen to a saturation target of 94%.

2. Take blood cultures and consider source control.

3. Administer empiric intravenous antibiotics.

4. Measure serial serum lactates.

5. Start intravenous fluid resuscitation.

6. Commence accurate urine output measurement.

Someone could argue that extremely sick patients, who are the ones who will require damage-control procedures, can be diagnosed on the spot by merely looking at them. They could also argue that a lot of scoring is useless and done only for scoring sake. We do not agree with them. It is imperative in our practice to assess the response to our treatment, and this can be done only if we have determined our starting point. We still use, as many other colleagues do, the concept and definitions of the "Surviving Sepsis Campaign: International Guidelines for the Management of Severe Sepsis and Septic Shock: 2012." We stress to our trainee the importance of assessing the patient and following their response to the treatment. Diagnosis at a glance also does not correlate with morbi-mortality, and it is not a common language used when dealing with other specialties, who would look upon your surgeon as a caveman.

We use the Sepsis definition, and the p-POSSUM score as a minimum to assess patient severity and surgical risk. We appreciate that P-POSSUM has been criticized, and possibly is not the best scoring tool available. Let us say that p-POSSUM is as bad as all the others available [7–9].

Septic patients are treated according to the Surviving Sepsis Campaign Bundle. Upon arrival, once the acute abdomen has been identified (again, it is a clinical diagnosis!), blood cultures are taken, and broad-spectrum antibiotics are started along with intravenous fluid replacement. For each hour of delay of antibiotic administration, there is a cumulative increase in mortality of 4%.

Which antibiotic should be administered is up to your hospital policies. Piperacillin/Tazobactam is the first choice in no-penicillin allergic patients in many hospitals.

Antibiotics, fluid, and oxygen are all you can do to start optimization and treatment. At the same time, you are now ready to pass the patient through the CT scan.

If you have done things correctly, you have lost no more than 30 min from arrival, and you should have been able to assess the problem (acute peritonitis), rule out other mimicking conditions (ruptured AAA clinically and laboratoristically is quite different) and evaluate the severity while starting the treatment. Ideally, a simple Chest X-ray should be performed during the initial assessment in the Accident & Emergency Department, to exclude free gas under the diaphragm (hollow viscous perforation). Furthermore, an abdominal ultrasound scan can exclude a AAA and give a piece of valuable information on possible free intraperitoneal fluid. Early involvement of a senior surgeon is crucial for the decision making and for coordinating with the other specialties.

An essential skill of the Emergency Surgeon should be interpreting CT scans. The Surgeon should be able to see the CT scan in real-time and seek advice from the Radiologist. Reviewing the scans together with the Radiologist, can give valuable information to the Surgeon and help him significantly to plan the strategy of the operation if needed. Since we are focusing on damage-control procedures, let us exclude all Hinchey I–II acute diverticulitis, and concentrate only on Hinchey III–IV, cases that are acute peritonitis. Usually, diagnosis of acute diffuse peritonitis is quite straightforward on a CT scan, even for a surgeon: free fluid, pneumoperitoneum, and fat stranding, alone or combined, are the key features. We see the CT scan, and we know that they will go to the OR for the source control.

Re-evaluation of the critically ill surgical patient is critical and essential. In many cases, the initial resuscitation has been adequate. The patient, hopefully, now has a good (or better) urinary output of at least 0.5 mL/Kg/h, is better perfused and does not require inotropic drugs. However, the patient still needs an emergency operation. In that case, the management options include a primary anastomosis with or without a prophylactic ileostomy or a Hartmann's procedure. That means that, most likely, a damage-control procedure is not needed.

Unfortunately, there are cases when the patient is not able to respond to resuscitation. The patient remains hypoperfused, oliguric/anuric, acidotic, coagulopathic, and often hypothermic. This sub-group of critically ill surgical patients is among the most challenging scenarios in emergency surgery. They are very often of old age, with multiple comorbidities and low reserves. They, unwillingly, form the vast majority of the mortality rate.

Yet, if you and the other members of the multidisciplinary team you are working with decide that invasive treatments are not futile, it is time to hurry up and do things properly.

In the real world, you have already spent at least 90 min: the patient has already been resuscitated all that it is advisable, and ideally, nothing can be added if source control is not obtained.

Just a couple of notes before entering the OR.

Remember the lethal triad in trauma: hypothermia, acidosis, and coagulopathy. We aim to fight those. Do not forget to actively warm your patients since they arrive to your observation. That means a warm environment and warm fluids. Also, if coagulation if deranged for the sepsis or in case they are on antiplatelet drugs or anticoagulants, you should involve the hematologist on-call as soon as possible, or use pre-existing protocols if available. It is not wise, although it is not infrequent, to find out an INR more than 2 just when you are ready to transfer them to OR. It is not a mortal sin, but it means more time to wait before source control, which, yes, increases mortality. Ways to correct the INR urgently in order to proceed with damage-control surgery include administering intravenous vitamin K, and transfusion of coagulation factor concentrates.

3. Operating room (OR)

Now the patients need a general anesthesia. Anesthetists know very well that the anesthetic management of these patients requires always a rapid sequence induction due to the high risk of bronchoaspiration.

This consists of giving the patient supplementary O_2 close to 100% for 30 s, asking to take three deep breaths as long as they are still conscious and collaborative. Subsequently, the hypnotic drug will be administered while another person assists by performing cricoid pressure. The cricoid pressure is maintained from the moment of induction until the intubation is completed. Applying pressure on the cricoid collapses the esophagus and prevents the passage of gastric contents to the larynx and respiratory tract. A fast-acting myorelaxant such as succinylcholine at a dose of 1 mg/kg iv or rocuronium at a dose of 1.2 mg/kg iv, will be administered just after the hypnotic drug. It will achieve a rapid opening of the vocal cords after approximately 15–20 s, allowing to pass the tracheal tube.

Basic intraoperative monitoring will be achieved by ECG, non-invasive TA, O_2 saturation by pulse oximetry, bispectral index (BIS), neuromuscular, core temperature, and hourly diuresis. Arterial canalization for invasive blood pressure monitoring and canalization is advised as well as obtaining a central venous route to administer large amounts of fluid therapy, vasopressors, blood products, or parenteral nutrition if required in the postoperative period [7, 10].

The primary anesthetic aim in these patients is to maintain or restore an adequate blood flow to guarantee an optimal O_2 delivery to the tissues. Objective-directed IV fluid therapy will be administered using dynamic hemodynamic variables (stroke volume variation—SVV, pulse pressure variation—PPV) to predict the response to fluid loading, guided by hemodynamic monitoring devices (CardioQ, PiCCo, and LiDCo) [11, 12]. If these devices were not available, static hemodynamic variables will be used with the following goals: maintaining central venous pressure >8 cm H_2O; mean arterial pressure (MAP) >65–70 mmHg; diuresis >0.5 ml/kg/h; a venous saturation central ($ScvO_2$) >70% or a mixed venous saturation of O_2 (SvO_2) >65 mmHg and normalization of lactate.

Unfortunately, static (HR, BP, and CVP) are not sensitive enough to predict a response to a fluid reposition and therefore are poor indicators of intravascular volume status.

Initial resuscitation with fluid therapy should be done with crystalloids. The administration of hydroxyethyl starch 130/0.4 should be avoided, as it appears to increase morbidity and mortality in these patients [13]. If the SSV or PPV are less than 10–15% with a PAM <65–70 mmHg despite the fluid challenge, or we do not have hemodynamic monitoring devices, but we have hypotension that does not respond to fluid therapy, vasopressors will be administered. Norepinephrine is the vasopressor of choice. Other options are adrenaline or vasopressin to reduce the dose of norepinephrine. Dobutamine will be administered in the presence of myocardial dysfunction or low cardiac output, or when signs of hypoperfusion persist despite adequate intravascular volume or MAP.

It is also necessary to maintain an adequate hydroelectrolytic and hemostatic balance, administering bicarbonate when essential and different hemostatic components to restore or maintain the coagulation. Coagulation can be assessed by standard tests, or by viscoelastic tests (VETs). The latter allow a treatment oriented assessment of coagulation, and if available should be used as first choice.

As for the transfusion of blood products, it is recommended to maintain hemoglobin levels between 7 and 9 g/dl, and glycemic levels should be kept below 180 mg/dl [14].

Now the ball is back in our court, the surgeon's.

Your patient is in a pretty bad clinical situation, and they will have a high mortality/morbidity rate whatever you are going to do. Your challenge is to make all the right decisions and quickly. Some of them are not straightforward, and will be surely discussed in the following M&M. Some are extremely easy though, and if you make mistakes here, you will be surely crucified in the M&M. So, for both the patient's sake and yours: do a laparotomy. If you are really convinced that laparoscopy is a good indication in a crashing patient in septic shock, you can as well stop reading this chapter, since you will not find anything useful for you.

We have too many hours of both elective laparoscopic colorectal surgery and emergency surgery to stand by what we are saying. Laparoscopy has no place in this scenario. So, prepare your OR for a formal laparotomy, with all the instruments you are going to need. We usually want advanced cautery devices in this case, as well as staplers, to minimize the OR time.

As we have already said, delaying the surgical procedure can lead to a progressive deterioration of the patient status, and it may contribute to a more unfortunate outcome.

The surgical team should be ready and prepared to operate even at night hours, because any delay is increasing the already high chances of losing the patient. Excellent communication and coordination between the attending team members should be emphasized; the team leader, generally, the surgeon should coordinate all the resources needed in order to complete the task swiftly. Well-organized teams formed by anesthetists, intensivists, and nursing staff will work faster and will obtain better results when a real team attitude is practiced.

Now that you are already scrubbed and about to start, keep in mind two easy concepts: size matters (big incision); time matters (be quick).

The key for a quick resection is good exposure: bone-to-bone midline laparotomy is just a few centimeters too long in this situation. Small incisions that compromise surgical exposure should be avoided. Proper retraction is also indispensable, self-retracting devices can be quite helpful, especially in obese patients. The abdominal wall should be protected with wall protectors that, in many cases, can be used both as protecting devices that reduce surgical site infection and also as an additional retracting tool.

Once the abdomen is opened, a quick general evaluation of the abdominal cavity should be routinely performed, and samples taken for aerobic and anaerobic cultures. The origin of the colonic wall perforation should be controlled temporarily by whatever means you fancy (clamps, sutures, staplers, etc.), and a first lavage should be carried out to remove gross contamination. Once this has been done, you will have to achieve a definitive source control, which can be done only by colonic resection (formal sigmoidectomy vs. segmental colectomy).

As a general rule, you will find extremely inflamed tissues, which, especially in obese patients, will make the dissection difficult. This is not a cancer operation, though. There is no need for you to go down in the mesentery to find the root of the inferior mesenteric artery (IMA) or the inferior mesenteric vein (IMV). You should be comfortable with the anatomy and the surgical technique and use judgment. This means that you should tailor the operation not only to the patient's needs, but also to your abilities. A proper retraction makes a lot of difference in difficult open surgery. If your assistant is more inexperienced than you and a more senior help is available, call them in: it is easy to operate when assisted by someone who knows how to.

The use of energy devices like the LigaSure Atlas of 10 mm–20 cm (Medtronic®) can be beneficial both for blunt dissection and also for hemostatic control of the thickened mesocolon, always taken care to identify the ureter in cases of sigmoid resection. The colonic segment should be excised using GIA reloadable stapling devices. After the resection is performed and the specimen extracted, a thorough washout of the abdominal cavity should be done with a warm saline solution with particular attention to the pouch of Douglas, left and right gutters, and both subphrenic areas.

The decision to whether performing a definitive procedure vs. a damage control should have already been taken before entering the OR since it should have been based on physiological assessment. It is improbable that after surgical aggression, the patient will be hemodynamically and physiologically better. In some rare circumstances though, you will find out that there are exceptions to what was stated before: the patient unexpectedly has significantly improved, maybe inotropes are being tapered down, urine output has normalized. In these circumstances, you can reconsider your previous decisions and go for a definitive procedure, namely primary anastomosis or terminal colostomy.

If we can give good-samaritan advice, twink twice, and then think once again. If you have access to modern systems for the open abdomen, you should not change your pre-op decision. We have all done it, and the results have not always been favorable. Be pragmatic and stick to doing damage-control, surgery.

In any case, the rule of the thumb is that you have been so quick (not kidding) that the anesthetists are still putting IV lines, and the patient is still unstable and on vasopressors. The surgical part of damage control is completed. We strongly advise to leave the stumps inside, perform a meticulous washout and leave a temporary abdominal closure for a second procedure in the following days, once the patient's conditions are more favorable for an anastomosis. Performing a stoma at this stage is time consuming, and really does not offer any advantage. Performing a primary anastomosis now, even if has been advocated by other colleagues, seems to us an unnecessary act. Our philosophy is to minimize the surgical aggression and the operative time.

If you have decided for a temporary closure of abdomen, you should already know that currently, there are several temporary abdominal closure devices available, and the use of one or another will depend on availability and the surgical team preference. One of the most used devices, and the one that we have more experience with, is the ABThera Sensa T.R.A.C ® (KCI) [1].

This is a temporary negative pressure abdominal closure therapy composed of four components. A visceral protective layer (VPL), a perforated foam, the plastic adherent drape, and tubing, connected a negative pressure source. These devices can help to protect the abdominal content and create a temporary functional abdominal closure avoiding a sustained or repeated pathologic elevation in abdominal pressure above 12 mmHg. Another benefit of the negative pressure therapy is that it actively removes fluid from the abdominal cavity and draws the wound edges together, avoiding fascial retraction. Both the initial application and subsequent dressing changes should be performed under aseptic conditions, either in the OR or in the ICU, between 24 and 72 h, depending on the level of contamination and infection of the abdominal cavity. With each dressing change, the surgical team should perform a thorough re-evaluation of the abdominal cavity and whether the abdomen can be finally closed, but the correct timing and the definitive closure should be individually tailored depending on the patient's general status and response to therapy.

These types of commercial devices have the advantage of delivering a controlled negative pressure throughout the abdominal cavity, especially in the paracolic gutters and pouch of Douglas, but they are expensive and not always available. In cases where there is no availability of these devices, then, an Barker closure of the abdomen can be done. It is similar to the one we use in trauma damage-control surgery. These improvised systems consist of using a layer that can cover the sensitive abdominal organs, and at the same time, keep them warm.

The layer can be made by two layers of surgical drape made with a robust, conformable, and breathable polyester incise film coated with medical-grade acrylate adhesive containing molecular iodine as the active antimicrobial agent. Between the layers, we use large swabs. After making the layer, we shape it and cut according to the gap we would like to cover. Because of the surgical drape that covers both sides, this layer can be inserted inside the abdomen and be in touch with the bowel without problems. Then, the whole abdomen (all four quadrants) is covered with an extra surgical drape offering adequate sealing. We need to highlight the need for insertion of two large abdominal drains (usually 30Fr) to drain potential intra-abdominal fluid and, most importantly, to prevent abdominal compartment syndrome.

4. Intensive care unit (ICU)

We surgeons have done what we could and had to do. The patients need now an Intensivist and an ICU. Your colleagues are expecting them to arrive at any time, the anesthetist has already called them, and everything is ready. Intensivists are well aware of what is at stake. They know that grade III and IV diverticulitis implies the presence of intestinal macro-perforations responsible for the appearance of purulent or fecaloid peritonitis, which is associated with a high percentage of complications such as peritoneal abscesses, pyogenic liver abscesses due to the dissemination of the process through the portal circulation, small intestine obstructions, fistulas, etc.

The most common germs are gram-negative bacilli such as enterobacteria, anaerobes, and less frequently Enterococci and *Pseudomonas aeruginosa*. In post-surgical patients, there is an increase in cases of *Staphylococcus aureus* infection resistant to methicillin and *Candida* sp. if they have received the previous antibiotherapy.

Secondary peritonitis can trigger a dysregulated response by our organism that can lead to sepsis or septic shock and multiorgan failure depending on the severity, which implies significant morbidity and mortality.

The recognition of a septic patient is based on the alteration of clinical and analytical parameters such as mean blood pressure (MAP) <70 mmHg or systolic pressure (SBP) <100 mmHg, renal failure with the presence of oliguria/anuria and increased creatinine levels >1.2 mg/dl, at the respiratory level may lead to respiratory distress syndrome that occurs with severe hypoxemia and need for respiratory support with high flow oxygen systems or invasive mechanical ventilation. Neurologically, obnubilation, or low level of consciousness may be seen. In terms of analytical parameters in the blood, metabolic acidosis, hyperlactacidemia, consumptive coagulopathy, and plaquetopenia stand out.

If the patient needs vasoactive substances after adequate volume replacement to maintain MAP >60 mmH and serum lactate is >2 mmol/l, it is called septic shock.

For treatment, from the first hours of admission, an attempt will be made to maintain adequate hemodynamic stability thanks to the administration of fluid therapy (30 ml/kg in the first 3 h) with intravenous crystalloids. The therapeutic and hemodynamic response will be re-evaluated frequently, to maintain Average Arterial Pension (MAP) >65 mmHg, Heart Rate (HR) >60, Oxygen Saturation (SO_2) >90%, Central Venous Pressure (CVP) 12–8 mmHg, Temperature <37°C, and Diuresis greater than 0.5 ml/kg/h. We will try to optimize different analytical parameters such as ions, renal function, liver function, lactate levels, presence of acidotic, alkaline or mixed pattern, platelet count, and hemoglobin, indicating the transfusion of red blood cells with hemoglobin levels ≤7 g/dL [15].

The lactic acid evaluated in a venous or arterial gasometry is a marker of adequate tissue irrigation, keeping our objectives in values lower than 2 mg/dL [15].

If, after initial resuscitation, the situation of instability persists, the initiation of vasopressors without delay is indicated, with Noradrenaline being the first-line agent in septic shock. In refractory cases, the start of other vasopressors such as vasopressin, inotropic agents such as dobutamine, and glucocorticoids may be indicated.

In the most severe cases, it will be necessary to implement different support measures such as renal replacement therapy, indicated in renal failure with oliguria or anuria and severe alteration of analytical values, invasive mechanical ventilation (IMV) in those who develop respiratory distress syndrome.

In these patients measurement of intra-abdominal pressure (IAP) is mandatory. If it exceeds 12 mmHg, we would speak of intra-abdominal hypertension and if it exceeds 20 mmHg of abdominal compartment syndromes with the need to use specific techniques such as placement of NGS, force negative balance. Since they already have a laparostomy it is unlikely, but not impossible, that they may need a further surgical decompression.

5. Back to OR

The operation has been done and the patient has been left in the experienced hands of ICU.

We do not fool ourselves: some (maybe many) of them will die in the next 12–24 h. The toll to pay is simply too much, especially in the case of elderly patients, or in the ones with many comorbidities. Usually the sicker, and more unstable, they were in theater, the sooner are expected to pass. We cannot give any percentage, because we do not have it, and also because it would be not pertinent to our story. Suffice to say that the reality is just a little better than what the P-POSSUM score told you, but not so much better as you would like.

For those who actually improve, they will eventually need a second operation, a so-called "second look."

The planning and decision making for a second look ideally were made by the operating surgeon while performing the initial damage-control surgical procedure. The second-look laparotomy is based on the fact that the surgeon should explore the patient's abdomen within 24 or 48 h, depending on the patient's hemodynamic stability. That means that a second-look laparotomy is a scheduled procedure and should ideally be performed in a patient that is stable with as less inotropic support as possible.

In any case, negative pressure abdominal dressings should be changed after 72 h most.

One of the most important parameters to have is the intra-abdominal pressure, or IAP. IAP should have been measured in ICU and you should prepare to measure it when attempting the closure.

Anesthetic-wise, usually the second-look poses no big challenges.

Intraoperatively, we have to assess if there is still contamination, the viability of the colonic stumps and whether or not there are any other issues that need to be dealt with (i.e., iatrogenic damages from the first surgery). Also, this is the time to finish the preparation of the proximal colon for the terminal colostomy.

In very selected cases, those who have improved very well in ICU and without comorbidities, we can opt for a primary anastomosis. Unfortunately, collectively, we have encountered very few of them. But we know that other colleagues have been more lucky.

Just a word about the rectal stump. It is quite uncommon to detect any problem at this level now, but not uncommon to have a dehiscence of the stump later on. We always leave a pelvic drain, only to drain the stump should it leak.

Usually, the "bowel" part of the second-look causes no big problem: whatever you do, it is more or less easy.

The challenge of the second-look is often the abdominal closure. Sometimes, it can be difficult to approximate the abdominal wound edges, mainly because of the edema of the intra-abdominal organs that can result in a high intra-abdominal pressure and difficulty to approximate the midline laparotomy edges successfully. The extent to which you can close the abdomen under tension is difficult to judge. We rely much on IAP, and feel safe to close if IAA is <12 mmHg. But also the quality of the tissue is crucial, and this is something that you cannot judge objectively.

As a rule, we do primary closure of the fascia is IAP <12 mmHg and accept the need of following surgeries for incisional hernia. We do not routinely do advanced abdominal wall reconstruction surgery at this stage, and prefer to do them, if indicated, during a former repair of an incisional hernia.

In the few cases, where you cannot close the abdomen due to elevated IAP, we use a **mesh-mediated** vacuum-assisted wound closure as proposed by Petersson et al., which in our hands is what works best [1].

An in-depth discussion of abdominal wall reconstruction is beyond the topic of this chapter.

Usually, after the second look, the patient will go back to the ICU. If the evolution is favorable in the following days, we can minimize the necessary support measures. In patients who have presented septic shock and multiorgan failure, we will progressively withdraw invasive mechanical ventilation, renal replacement therapies, and vasoactive drugs, depending on the recovery of these organs.

It is essential after overcoming the initial shock situation, at 24–48 h, to initiate adequate nutritional therapy since patients in septic shock suffer a hypercatabolic phase mediated by increased cytokines and lipid mediators with a peak between 3 and 4 days but which can be maintained for 7–10 days.

6. Conclusions

Whether you are an experienced (old) surgeon, an enthusiastic (not quite old) fellow, or a young trainee, you will be facing, again and again, patients with acute diverticulitis. When called upon to assess them, you will know beforehand that most of them will be Hinchey I–II, and commonly only a small number of them will have diffuse peritonitis, purulent, or fecal. As an experienced clinician, you should be assessing the patient's physiologic status even before considering whether your patient has acute diverticulitis or other conditions. Early in your evaluation, you should determine whether you are dealing with septic but contained infection or a patient with septic shock. Patients with sepsis should be treated promptly and appropriately to avoid fatal outcomes.

Currently, the application of the Sepsis-Six protocol is indicated, and it should be applied as soon as possible. This approach implies being very aggressive in management. It is advisable to start resuscitation even before having made a diagnosis of the cause. Once you have started your resuscitation and treatment based on your clinical experience, you can confirm your findings with blood-test results and imaging studies in cases of sepsis due to severe acute diverticulitis the CT scan (always with IV contrast) will provide you with valuable information.

If you have done things correctly, you will not only have diagnosed the etiology but also, and most importantly, you will have a diagnosis of severity. Sepsis due to acute diverticulitis with diffuse peritonitis without septic shock or contained is not the same as "unresponsive" septic shock due to the same condition. There is a massive difference in morbidity and mortality among both presentations. When in shock, all the derangement of the physiological status and its response to resuscitation should not be delayed. If you wait to complete the work-up and delay initial treatment, you will waste precious time and have an unfavorable outcome and higher mortality.

You should follow your clinical instinct and make a correct initial evaluation, anticipating the needs of your patient, and preparing your team approach. Surgeons, anesthetists, radiologists, OR nurses, are all part of this team and should be prepared. For those patients with unresponsive septic shock, consider damage-control as the approach that will maximize the possibility of recovery to your patient. Imagine a patient with an unresponsive septic shock as a KO-ed boxer. He needs to stop the fight, has his opponent removed from the ring, and be allowed to rest and recover before being able to fight another match and maybe win it. Damage-control is removing the opponent (source control) and resting and recovering (ICU). Even if there are no guarantees, your patient may return to fight another day. In our scenario, it is all about doing a quick source control followed by resuscitation in ICU, leaving the definitive procedure for when your patient is in a better physiological status.

Your team of clinicians formed by the surgeon, anesthetist, intensivist, knows how to do it.

As an experienced surgeon, remember that is not the patient for a key-hole surgical approach. It is mandatory to have good exposure and to be quick: nothing less than a good (almost)-full midline laparotomy is advisable. Surgery should be easy; try not to complicate it yourself: non-oncological resection with stapler, leave everything inside, do a temporary closure of the abdomen and come back after 24–48 h if the patient survives.

A final word for the forgotten actors of this play: the patient and their family. We are not going to linger on the consent form or other bureaucratic matters. We want to stress that they should be kept involved in the decision process and also be informed frankly on the expected timeline. People do not quickly grasp the concept of open abdomen and second look. The standard expectation for surgical treatment is not to start today and finish after 2 or 3 days if all goes well. The information you give to them and honest expectations are critical in these complex scenarios. So, try to be consensual with your colleagues and avoid discrepancies in the information provided; this maintains the patients' and family members' trust in the assisting team. Sometimes you have to sit down again and again and go through everything you have already explained with your patient and family members.

You should provide not only surgical techniques and medications but also provide support to the worried families as well. Sometimes they only need some empathy and a word of comfort, or just feeling that you (or whoever is in charge) cares about their dear ones. Taking time to give your support and listen to the patient and his family's concerns is never a waste of time.

Author details

Luca Ponchietti[1*], Néstor Bueno Vidales[1], Andrea A. Casamassima[2], Fernando Gallego Estrada[1], Alessandro Garcea[3], Ioannis Gerogiannis[4], Alberto Lafita López[1], Diego Mariani[5], Olga Marin Casajús[1], Matteo Marconi[6], Nuno Filipe Muralha Antunes[7], Laura María Pradal Jarne[8], Jorge Vera Bella[1] and Carlos Yánez Benítez[9]

1 Hospital San Jorge, Huesca, Spain

2 ASST Melegnano e della Martesana, PO Santa Maria delle Stelle, Melzo, Milano, Italy

3 Hospital Universitario de Elche, Elche, Spain

4 Kingston Hospital NHS Foundation Trust, London, United Kingdom

5 ASST OVEST MILANESE, Legnano, Italy

6 ASST-Ovest Milanese Po Fornaroli Magenta, Magenta, Italy

7 Centro Hospitalar Médio Ave, Santo Tirso/Famalicão, Portugal

8 Hospital Clínico Universitario Lozano Blesa, Zaragoza, Spain

9 Hospital Royo Villanova, Zaragoza, Spain

*Address all correspondence to: lponchietti@salud.aragon.es

References

[1] Petersson U, Acosta S, Björck M. Vacuum-assisted wound closure and mesh-mediated fascial traction—A novel technique for late closure of the open abdomen. World Journal of Surgery. 2007;**31**(11):2133-2137

[2] Sartelli M, Catena F, Ansaloni L, Coccolini F, Griffiths EA, Abu-Zidan FM, et al. WSES Guidelines for the management of acute left sided colonic diverticulitis in the emergency setting. World Journal of Emergency Surgery: WJES. 2016;**11**:37

[3] Andeweg CS, Mulder IM, Felt-Bersma RJ, et al. Guidelines of diagnostics and treatment of acute left-sided colonic diverticulitis. Digestive Surgery. 2013;**30**(4-6):278-292. DOI: 10.1159/000354035

[4] Feingold D, Steele SR, Lee S, Kaiser A, Boushey R, Buie WD, et al. Practice parameters for the treatment of sigmoid diverticulitis. Diseases of the Colon and Rectum. 2014;**57**:284-294

[5] Hong MKY, Tomlin AM, Hayes IP, Skandarajah AR. Operative intervention in acute diverticulitis. ANZ Journal of Surgery. 2015;**85**:734-738. DOI: 10.1111/ans.13126

[6] Cirochchi R et al. A historical review of surgery for peritonitis secondary to acute colonic diverticulitis: From Lockhart-Mummery to evidence-based medicine. World Journal of Emergency Surgery. 2017;**12**:14

[7] Rhodes A, Evans L, et al. Surviving sepsis campaign: International Guidelines for management of sepsis and septic shock. Critical Care Medicine Journal. 2017;**45**:3

[8] Gaieski DF, Mikkelsen ME. Evaluation of and initial approach to the adult patient with hypotension and shock. UpToDate. [Accessed on April 2020]. Available from: https://www.uptodate.com/contents/evaluation-of-and-initial-approach-to-the-adult-patient-with-undifferentiated-hypotension-and-shock

[9] Schmidt GA, Mandel J. Evaluation and management of suspected sepsis and shock in adults. UpToDate. [Accessed on April 2020]. Available from: https://www.uptodate.com/contents/evaluation-and-management-of-suspected-sepsis-and-septic-shock-in-adults/print

[10] Ortega D, Narváez L, Valencia C, Cisneros M, Hernández Z, Zúñiga A. Anestesia en el paciente séptico. Revista Chilena de Anestesia. 2019;**48**(3):230-239

[11] Kelm DJ, Perrin JT, Carlin-Ceba R, Galic O, Schenck L, Kennedy CC. Fluid overload in patients with severe sepsis and septic shock treated with early goal-directed therapy is associated with increased acute need for fluid-related medical interventions and hospital death. Shock. 2015;**43**(1):68-73

[12] Grupo de Trabajo de la Vía Clínica de Recuperación Intensificada en Cirugía Abdominal. Vía Clínica de Recuperación Intensificada en Cirugía Abdominal (RICA). Ministerio de Sanidad, Servicios Sociales e Igualdad e Instituto Aragonés de Ciencias de la Salud; 2014. NIPO: 680-15-085-5. Available from: https://www.mscbs.gob.es/gl/biblioPublic/publicaciones.do?metodo=detallePublicacion&publicacion=11170

[13] Annane D, Fuchs-Buder T, Zoellner C, Kaukonen M, Scheeren TWL. EMA recommendation to suspend HES is hazardous. [published correction appears in Lancet. 2018 Mar 10;**391**(10124):e8]. Lancet. 2018;**391**(10122):736-738. DOI:10.1016/S0140-6736(18)30254-X

[14] Irwin RS, Rippe JM. Procedures, Techniques and Minimally Invasive Monitoring in Intensive Care Medicine. 4th ed. Philadelphia: Wolters Kluwer Health; 2008

[15] Puppo Moreno AM, Abella Alvarez A, Morales Conde S, Perez Flecha M, Garcia Ureña MÁ. La unidad de cuidados intensivos en el postoperatorio de cirugía mayor abdominal. Medicina Intensiva. 2019;**45**(3):569-577

Chapter 6

Diagnosis and Treatment of Midface Trauma in the Context of Polytrauma: Characteristics during COVID-19 Pandemic Conditions

Daniela Vrinceanu, Bogdan Banica and Mihai Dumitru

Abstract

Midfacial trauma is never an immediate therapeutic emergency excepting cases with nasal bleeding and risk of aspiration or requiring a permeable airway that will allow intubation when appropriate. The patient with polytraumas and midfacial fractures who needs ear, nose, and throat (ENT) or oral and maxillofacial (OMF) surgery should be reassessed at 24 and 48 hours to determine the optimal operating time. The surgical indication should be established according to esthetic and functional deficits. We consider that the optimal operative moment for the lesions of the midface is at 4–5 days after the trauma, under the conditions of a stable hemodynamic, respiratory, and afebrile patient. We propose the schematic presentation of the principles of diagnosis and treatment for midface trauma. We will discuss also some aspects of midfacial trauma during coronavirus disease-2019 (COVID-19) pandemic conditions. We must assume every patient with polytrauma as a COVID-19-positive patient. So, it is necessary to have a special circuit for a suspect COVID-19 polytrauma patient between emergency room (ER) department, operating room, and intensive care unit (ICU). All medical team must wear high-level personal protective equipment (PPE) during emergency treatment of a craniofacial trauma in the context of polytrauma until we get the result of RT-PCR testing.

Keywords: face, trauma, diagnosis, treatment, COVID-19

1. Introduction

Trauma at the level of the head and neck represents a public health problem due to the esthetic and functional complications with major social and economic impacts. Among the possible causes for trauma stand car accidents, domestic violence, work-associated accidents, and even terrorist attacks [1].

These cases often have a legal consequence, and in this aspect, the ear, nose, and throat (ENT) surgeon represents a source of medical information important in establishing the degree of judiciary responsibility. The ENT surgeon must bear this in mind and keep accurate records of the procedures performed. Also different

 IntechOpen

pathologies before trauma along with alcohol consumption and high-risk drug intoxication are mentioned [2].

Photographically documenting the case before and after surgical procedures with subsequent electronic storage for later use is particularly important. In each department, there should be a person assigned to archiving images in potential legal and scientific cases of interest associating tumors or deep neck infections with the patient's death [3].

Patients with multiple trauma lesions admitted to the emergency department undergo assessment according to the ABCDE algorithm: A, airway plus spinal cord control; B, breath and ventilation; C, circulation and hemorrhage control; D, disability/neurologic status; and E, complete exposure but preventing hypothermia [4].

Facing a patient with multiple trauma lesions, a thorough head-to-toe lesion inventory with additional consults performed by the abdominal surgeon, thoracic surgeon, orthopedic surgeon, and others is necessary. For the head lesions, opinions from the neurosurgeon, ENT surgeon, OMF surgeon, ophthalmologist, and plastic surgeon should be gathered. The central pawn in this endeavor is the emergency specialist in the first stage and afterward the anesthesiologist supervising the case in the intensive care unit (ICU). Other lesions have a priority before facial fractures unless there is massive nasal bleeding with cerebrospinal fluid (CSF) leak or lesions hindering the oral intubation for general anesthesia. In the first case, the ENT surgeon must perform emergency nasal packing and in the other scenario must submit the patient to an emergency tracheostomy [5].

2. Principles of diagnosis in craniofacial trauma in cases with multiple trauma

The diagnosis must be correct and complete without the pressure of emergency, life-threatening bleeding, or from the patient's relatives or even other surgical specialties. After stopping any nasal bleeding and securing airway patency, perform head and neck computed tomography (CT) scan [6].

While performing the clinical examination in head trauma cases, pay attention to important nasal pyramid deviations, abnormal motility of the maxillary, trismus, facial hematomas surrounding both orbital regions, and exophthalmia. Especially important is vision assessment performed by the ophthalmologist. The clinical examination should be performed in a gentle but secure fashion with a predefined succession of maneuvers from the upper third of the face downward and ending with visualizing the nasal and oral cavities [7].

Do not forget to assess the presence of blood in the ear canal because it could be a sign of skull base fracture. ENT endoscopy should be reserved for the 24- to 48-hour follow-up to confirm the presence of a nasal cerebrospinal fluid leak. CSF leak is confirmed also through a lab workup by collecting the seeping clear fluid in a sterile recipient and looking for beta-transferrin levels [8].

Head CT scan in axial and coronal sections is compulsory, but frequently sagittal section reconstructions offer useful data about the anterior segment of the skull base and orbital floor. 3D reconstructions are useful for surgical planning and even explaining the patient the complexity of the trauma and improve informed consent (**Figure 1**) [9].

While formulating the complete diagnosis of cranial and facial trauma, one must take into consideration the various classification systems, imaging data, and even the cause and mechanism of trauma production. There are still limitations in

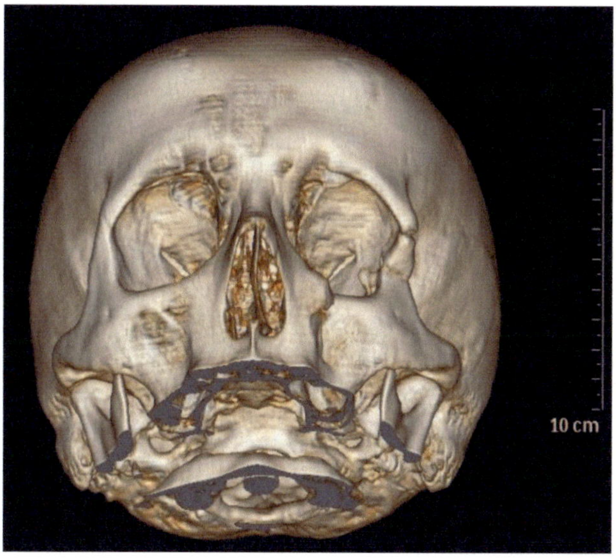

Figure 1.
CT scan with a complex maxillary-orbital-zygomatic fracture on the left side.

prediction with high accuracy of the functional and esthetic outcomes of the case. Afterward, perform a complete inventory of the other trauma lesions [10].

2.1 Classification of midfacial fractures according to LeFort

In 1901 LeFort described the midfacial fracture types I, II, and III after previous experimentally induced models. This classification is in use even nowadays because it is practical in nature and enables a common language between the trauma specialists. Often fracture lines are not complete bilaterally but still enable correct assessment of middle vault head trauma [11].

Low-transverse fracture LeFort type I has a direct mechanism of production through frontal and lateral impact or indirect by applying pressure in the mental region with the mouth closed. Fracture lines begin in the lower third of the nasal vault, above the dental roots through the canine fossa, along the zygomatic ridge through the maxillary tuberosity, and the lower third of the pterygoid. Also, there could be two possible scenarios with fixed or mobile fragments [12].

The clinical facial exam is scarce. The oral cavity presents chemosis in the labial groove and oral vestibule with dental occlusion dysfunctions and specific pain-triggering points behind the third molar teeth on the external pterygoid plate. In the case of a mobile fractured fragment, there is a supplementary fracture line in the vomer bone. Therefore, the physical examination will record the upper mobile alveolar bone along with the hard palate [13].

Middle-level transverse fracture LeFort type II presents a direct mechanism of production through a frontal impact in the middle vault of the viscerocranium. Fracture lines begin in the middle third of the nasal opening through the nasal bones bilaterally, the ascending arch of the maxillary bone, the lacrimal bone, the ethmoid bone, the floor of the orbit till the spheno-maxillary junction, the anterior wall of the maxillary sinus, and the middle third of the pterygoid plate [14].

The physical examination is marked by the presence of marked swelling of the face, inferior eyelid chemosis with epiphora, depression of anteroposterior facial landmarks with preservation of the zygomatic bones, depression of the nasal bones, nasal

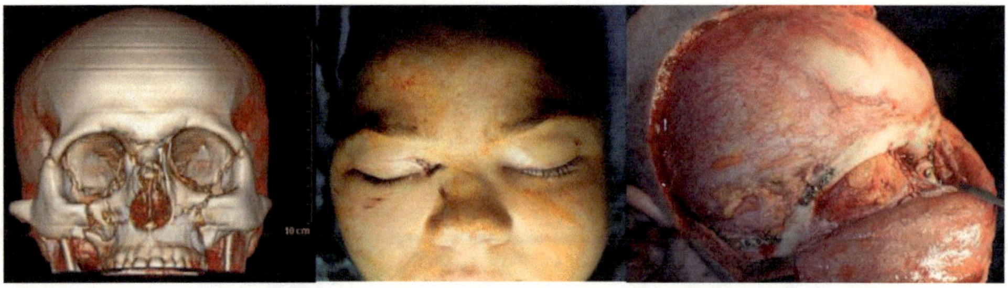

Figure 2.
Fracture LeFort type III—CT scan with 3D reconstruction, clinical aspect before surgery, and surgical reconstruction with titanium plates.

bleeding, subcutaneous emphysema, and infraorbital grove numbness. The oral cavity exam shows swelling of the superior vestibule, dental occlusion difficulties in vertical and sagittal planes, maxillary depression, and lack of lateral teeth superposition [15].

High-level transverse fracture LeFort type III has a violent mechanism of production at the level of the glabella or from lateral. The trajectory of such a fracture passes through the vomer, upper third of the nasal bones, ascending arch of the maxillary, ethmoid bone, floor of the orbit, external orbital wall, upper third of the pterygoid plate, and zygomatic arch [16].

At physical examination, the case presents depression of the nasal vault, tumefaction around both orbits, blood in the anterior eye pole, nasal bleeding, double vision, and facial subcutaneous emphysema. The oral cavity exam shows an abnormal movement in vertical and transverse planes of the mandible with retrognate maxillary bone and abnormal teeth occlusion (**Figure 2**) [17].

An emergency CT scan is compulsory in both axial and coronal planes with 3D reconstructions extremely helpful in planning surgery [18].

2.2 Classification of fractures of the middle facial vault according to the bones involved

There are nasal fractures, combined nasal-orbital-ethmoid fractures, and complex maxillary-orbital-zygomatic fractures. This classification has a clinical importance and eases communication between clinicians [19].

2.3 Classification of midfacial fractures given the impact energy

From this point of view, we encounter fractures with high energy and low energy. So, the diagnosis should include the landmarks in the midface affected according to the clinical exam, along with the information provided by the CT scan and ideally visualizing pretreatment 3D reconstructions [20].

3. Principles of treatment in craniofacial multiple trauma cases

3.1 Preliminary data

First, we have to secure the airway. Then, control nasal bleeding and other hemorrhages at the level of head and neck (**Figure 3**). Exclude any lesion at the level of the cervical spine. Also, check for any other occult life-threatening lesions such as spleen ruptures. This implies a second top-to-toe complete evaluation in 48 hours from the admission time and before any surgical interventions at the level

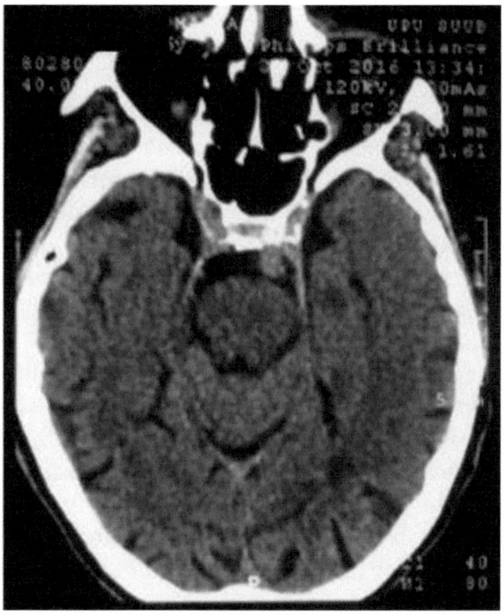

Figure 3.
CT scan performed for a nasal vault concussion without fracture of the nasal bones but with a fracture at the level of the ethmoid perpendicular plate associated with CSF leak (accidental fall on the stairs).

of the head and neck along with a complete inventory of all the lesions presented by the patient. Moreover, question the patient if possible or the relatives about prior associated pathology which could have an essential role in the prognosis and treatment outcome [21].

3.2 Clinical signs requiring a dynamic evaluation in the early stage of admission

Some clinical signs are requiring recurrent analysis during the early time of admission of multiple trauma patients: state of consciousness or drowsiness, increase in facial hematomas, increase pressure in orbital hematomas, high fever, the appearance of CSF at the level of the nasal cavity or the external ear canal, double vision, aggravation of mastication impairment, and loss of sensitivity in trigeminal nerve territory [22].

3.3 Treatment plan in craniofacial trauma cases

This sequence of steps should focus on repairing all the lesions with full restoration of function and the esthetic aspect before the trauma. The therapy plan should focus initially on clinical signs and secondarily on the CT exam. Global management of the case should benefit from the input of various specialists such as ICU specialists, anesthesia specialists, and surgeons from all other backgrounds available in the healthcare unit on call. Recent photos of the patient along with dental X-rays before trauma may be useful in lesion assessment and clear future legal aspects. Surgical interventions may be postponed due to increasing facial hematomas, nasal CSF leak, high fever, and thoracic concussions [23].

3.4 Specific considerations regarding the midface trauma

In cases with severe deformity, our experience recommends avoiding a conservative approach via small multiple regional "conservative/cosmetic" incisions. For a successful outcome, it is best to achieve a complete regional exposure through a coronal or hemicoronal flap (**Figure 4**) combined with a lower eyelid or intraoral incision if necessary [24].

The reduction of the zygomatic bone is best achieved via an intraoral vestibular approach as opposed to a temporalis approach, due to the loosening of the periosteum over the anterior surface of the maxilla and zygomatic buttress. Also, it allows sinus cavity exploration, evacuation of the sinus hematoma with an antiseptic irrigation, and, if necessary, plating along the maxilla-zygomatic buttress [25].

In orbital floor reconstruction, the reconstruction material should extend posteriorly to the orbital ridge of the palatine bone with a slight upward contour. A short, inferiorly inclined plate leads to persistent hypoglobus. In large orbital floor defects, we believe that it is important to avoid using other alloplastic materials than titanium due to the risk of globe mispositioning and possible local inflammatory response due to lack of rigid fixation and mobility (**Figure 5**) [26].

Do not delay the surgical intervention for more than 14 days. Except in a few numbers of severe polytrauma cases, the general condition of the patient should be stabilized in this time frame, and definitive treatment should be undertaken. After 14 days the case must follow the protocol of secondary reconstruction, because of the consolidation of the fractures and the treatment is incomparably more difficult [27].

3.5 Nasal bone fractures

These fractures require closure early within 24–48 hours except the cases with massive facial swelling and presenting nasal CSF leak. A clinical examination of the modified aspect of the nasal vault should be completed with plain X-ray of the nasal bones. Bear in mind the risk of secondary skull base fractures appearing during maneuvers for closing the nasal fracture. From the beginning of this chapter, we emphasized the importance of photos before and after the surgical procedure to prevent subsequent legal actions [28].

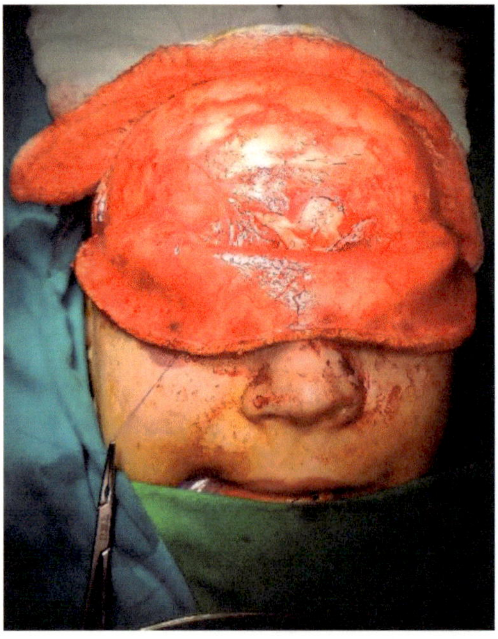

Figure 4.
Coronal approach for a complex nasal-orbital-ethmoid fracture.

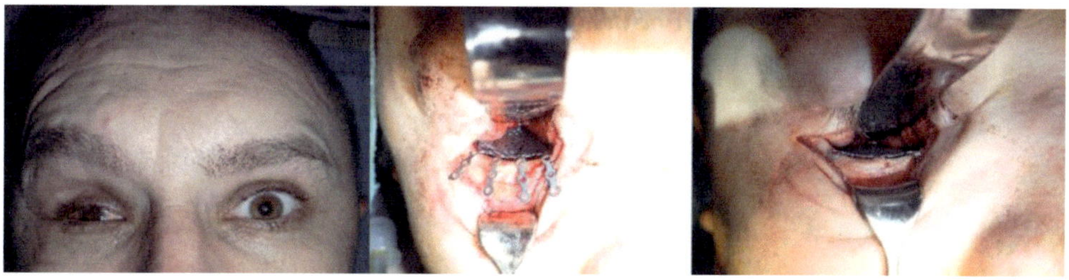

Figure 5.
Clinical aspect before surgery in a case with trauma on the right side with unfunctional eyeball—reconstruction of the orbit floor with a modified titanium mesh for sustaining the artificial eye prosthesis introduced subsequently.

General anesthesia is compulsory to relax the muscles and gain comfort for both the patient and the surgical team. Performing any maneuver on a shocked patient is forbidden. In cases of multiple fractures, the surgery may be scheduled in 4–5 days to give time for all the edema to resolute. A nasal fracture forms a callus in 8–10 days, so closed reduction is viable because the bones are still mobile in the fracture site during this time frame [29].

Open reduction of the fractures is reserved only for specific cases such as open fractures with fragments penetrating the skin or in cases of animal attacks requiring rabies or antitetanic treatment. The surgical steps will focus on direct closure of the fracture site with or without metal plates, nasal packing, and the reconstruction of tissues and sutures. Preserving the fracture site is obtained by both internal nasal packing and external metal splint placing [30].

3.6 Nasal-orbital-ethmoid complex fractures

These are overly complex fractures in the midface compartment with possible serious consequences from an esthetic and functional point of view. These cases frequently present a CSF leak. Clinically a quite easy assessment of the suspicion of a CSF leak is performed by observing the appearance of a pink hallow around the nasal blood droplets collected on a clean tissue [31].

Moreover, the persistent nasal bleeding should raise the question of a nasal CSF leak. Panda eyes sign of orbital hematomas is frequently associated with nasal CSF leak. In these cases, it is compulsory to perform a nasal endoscopy in the first 24 hours from the trauma to exclude CSF leak (**Figure 6**) [32].

When suspecting a CSF leak, we must postpone surgical closure of the nasal vault fractures because the maneuvers can aggravate the lesions in the skull base. The CT scan confirms the fractures at the level of the nasal and ethmoid bones [33].

Consequently, imaging studies should gather data in all three axial planes with thin slices and 3D reconstructions (**Figure 7**). Particularly useful is close cooperation with the radiologist to perform serial images of the skull base and visualize the associated lesions of the lacrimal sack. In this type of fractures, open reduction after the resolution of edema under general anesthesia is recommended (**Figure 8**) [34].

3.7 Principles of osteosynthesis (internal fixation) in midface trauma

The general principles of osteosynthesis were formulated in 1958 by the Association for Osteosynthesis (AO) and are the guidelines for osteosynthesis. The principles of osteosynthesis in midface trauma respect general principles, and they are as follows:

- **Rigid fixation**—rigid fixation will produce a three-dimensional stability of the fracture site, promoting primary fracture healing. The healing is extremely susceptible to mechanical influences. Mobility at the fracture site is one of the main causes of healing disturbances, and stability is considered the best protection against fracture site contamination and malunion [35].

- **Preservation of blood supply**—it is achieved by gentle handling and reduction of bone and soft tissue and by careful cold irrigation during the drilling phase, which must be performed at low rotation less than 1500 rpm to prevent the overheating of the bone structures. Good-quality instruments and osteosynthesis materials are mandatory [36].

- **Anatomical reduction/repositioning**—one must achieve anatomical correct repositioning of all midfacial bones. The height, width, and projection must be reestablished. The fracture lines must be surgically exposed and reduced before osteosynthesis [37].

- **Early mobilization**—early mobilization of the operated area and the patient allows a functional aftercare [38].

3.8 Medical treatment in cranial-facial trauma

3.8.1 Antibiotics

The treatment scheme should include third-generation cephalosporins, along with metronidazole due to oral bacteria contamination. This association of antibiotics has many advantages: it covers the spectrum of gram-positive bacteria encountered in ENT practice and also anaerobic bacteria and penetrates the blood–brain barrier [39].

These should be administered for at least 48 hours during nasal packing but better for 5–7 days including surgery and up to 14 days in cases with nasal CSF leaks. Meropenem or carbapenems after discussing with the neurosurgeon in cases with brain lesions or following local treatment protocols are also associated [40].

3.8.2 Corticoids

In this case, the neurosurgeon may prevent administering these compounds due to cerebral trauma. But for other lesions at the level of the viscerocranium, corticoids are beneficent reducing facial swelling and edema along the cranial nerve

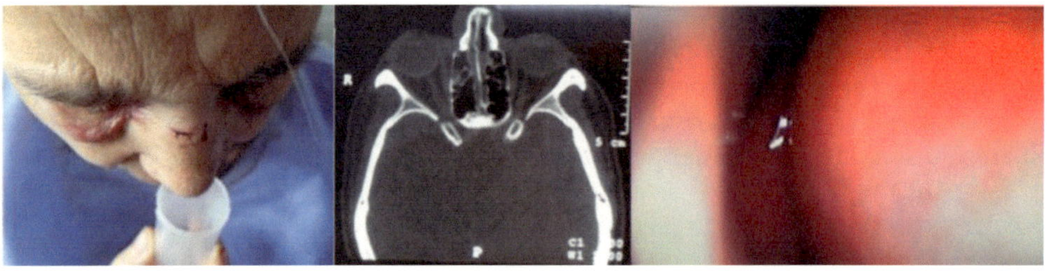

Figure 6.
Combined fracture of nasal vault and septum with CSF leak on the left side—clinical aspect, CT scan revealing fracture lines through the nasal septum and left nasal bone, also the endoscopic aspect of the CSF leak in a case with accidental fall from the same level.

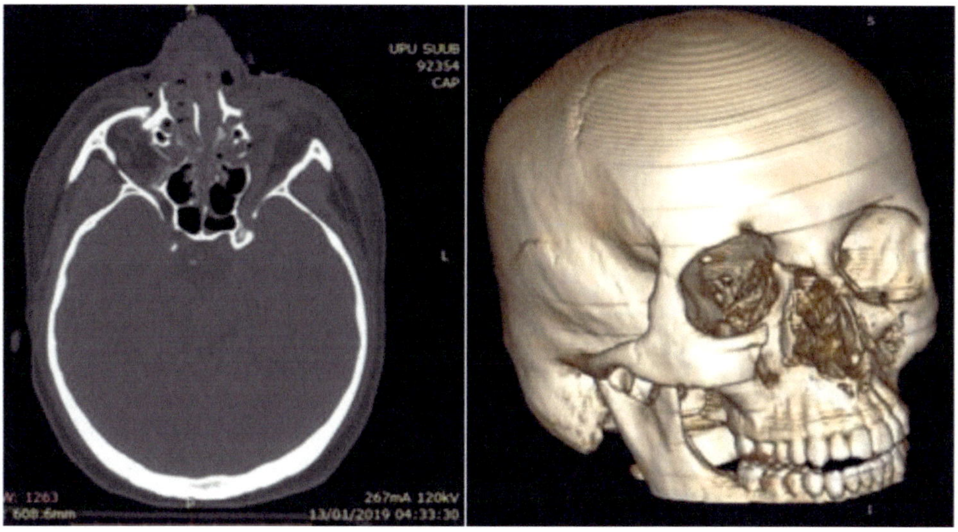

Figure 7.
A complex fracture involving the nasal vault, orbit, and ethmoid in axial section and 3D reconstruction imaging.

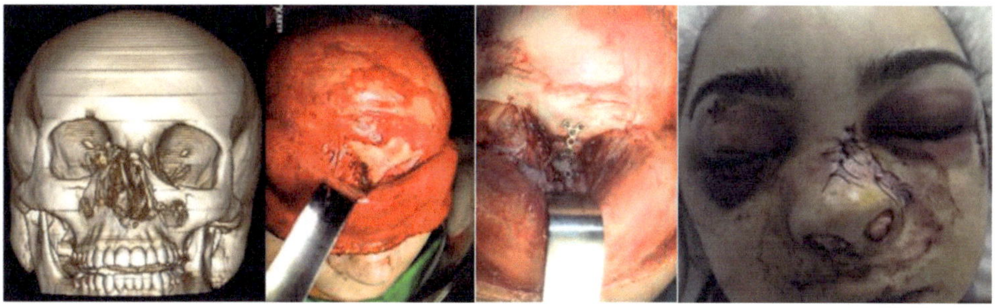

Figure 8.
A complex fracture involving the nasal vault, orbit, and ethmoid bone—CT scan with 3D reconstruction, surgical aspects of the coronal approach, and closing the fracture with titanium plates mounted in a Y pattern and final aspect at the end of the surgical procedure.

endings and preventing major functional deficits completely assessed many days after the trauma [41].

Such situations are facial palsy with inner ear lesions or eyesight impairment due to indirect compression or elongation of the optic nerve. Sometimes efficient corticoid regimens can even reduce the need for surgical treatment [42].

3.8.3 Analgesics

Painkillers from various classes may be used ranging from paracetamol to non-steroids and opioids or morphine if the patient is transferred to ICU with the help and continuous adjustment of the anesthesia and pain specialist [43].

3.8.4 Gastric secretion modulators

These compounds are proton pump inhibitors used to diminish the impact of traumatic stress and because of lack of oral food intake in the first 24 hours, but also to control the interactions between corticoids and analgesic compounds [44].

Other treatments in managing midfacial trauma include the following:

- **Early removal of nasal packing in the first 24 hours** enables clearing the paranasal sinuses of blood clots [45].

- **Nasal sprays** enable correct daily cleaning of the nasal cavity and drainage of secretions [46].

- **Vitamins B** are useful for preserving neural functions affected by trauma [47].

- **Injectable vitamin C** in high quantity quickens the resolution of facial swelling [48].

- **Psychological support** is compulsory in head and neck trauma cases, and the attending surgeon and specialized clinical psychologist should be involved or even psychiatric support in self-inflicted lesions [49].

3.9 Indication of surgical treatment in craniofacial trauma

Surgical treatment should focus on functional and esthetic deficits. Regarding early intervention in facial trauma, neurosurgeons consider the risks greater than the benefits. Therefore, surgery in these cases should be scheduled within 4–7 days to enable remission of edema and patient stabilization [50].

An exception from this rule is nasal bone fractures which require reduction within the first 24–48 hours from the accident to prevent secondary skull base fractures. We emphasized previously that this is possible under general anesthesia along with solving other fractures within 4–5 days from trauma [51].

Given the presence of CSF leak, the surgery must be postponed, and surgical reduction of fractures is possible within 10 days without a major change of the outcome [52].

4. Management of cranial-facial trauma in the context of COVID-19 pandemics

Trauma is an emergency pathology requiring urgent admission with quick analysis and treatment even in the context of current SARS-COV2 pandemics. Therefore, each hospital must establish a clear circuit of the patient from presentation to emergency distribution, operating room, and designated ICU compartment [53].

Cases with multiple traumas must be considered a highly COVID-19 suspect case, and the medical personnel attending the patient should wear level 3 personal protective equipment (PPE). These cases require testing with both rapid serological tests for SARS-COV2 and nasopharynx swab for RT-PCR testing before any maneuver in the emergency department [54].

In cases requiring CPR, the protocol has changed requiring paramedics to wear at least level 2 PPE and to restrain from performing external cardiac compressions and mouth-to-mouth breathing. These maneuvers should be performed by designated personnel equipped according to the national guidelines. The ENT and OMF surgeon is solicited in emergency cases with nasal bleeding, cases with difficult intubation due to neck-associated trauma, or mandible complex fractures. Regardless of the type of emergency, the ENT or OMF surgeon must be equipped with high-level PPE due to the high risk of contamination with SARS-COV2 attending trauma patients [55].

After examining the fractures, the patient is often transferred directly into the operating room allotted to COVID-19 cases due to its still uncertain virologic status. A major problem is that the results from the RT-PCR test are available only after some hours in the best-case scenario if not even the next day in some medical facilities. The operating room assigned for COVID-19 suspects must be isolated from operating rooms used in other elective surgeries. Following the example of Singapore, this operating room should be remotely placed and equipped with negative air pressure if possible. Moreover, it should be equipped with designated mobile imaging equipment. The access circuit in this operating theater should be specially designed and prevent cross-contamination of patients and personnel. The surgery should be performed with level 3 PPE equipment for the entire staff.

From the operating room, the patient is taken to the ICU specially designed for the COVID-19 suspect cases until obtaining the results of the RT-PCR test.

If the result of the test is negative, the patient will be transferred to the ICU designated for non-COVID cases and undergo the management of a usual multiple trauma victim. Craniofacial fractures need reassessment after 48 hours according to the previously stated guidelines. If the result of the RT-PCR is positive, the case needs to be stabilized and transferred to a designated COVID-19 support hospital. In this case, an examination of an infectious disease specialist is also necessary.

The current COVID-19 pandemics changes the type of emergency healthcare provided considering any trauma case as positive from the very beginning and requiring all personnel to wear level 3 PPE along with allotting separate diagnosis and treatment circuits with a reduced number of doctors but highly trained and referral as quickly as possible toward the COVID-19 designated healthcare facility for further management.

5. Conclusions

In complex cases with severe deformity, avoid a conservative approach via small multiple regional "conservative" incisions. For a successful outcome, it is best to achieve a complete regional exposure through a coronal or hemicoronal flap combined with lower eyelid or intraoral incision if necessary. Do not delay the surgical intervention for more than 14 days. Except in a few numbers of severe polytrauma cases, the general condition of the patient should be stabilized in this time frame, and definitive treatment should be undertaken. After 14 days the case has to follow the protocol of secondary reconstruction, because of the consolidation of the fractures and the treatment is incomparably more difficult. Do not evaluate the CT scan only in the axial view. For a complete assessment, it is mandatory to examine the CT scan in coronal, frontal, and 3D reconstruction views. If the clinical signs are not convergent with the CT scan interpretation, or if the fractures visible on the CT scan are associated with very little or no functional deficit, the "wait-and-see" or "conservative" approach should be taken into consideration, with the focus on glucocorticoid treatment. Surgical techniques should be tailored taking into consideration the functional and esthetic deficits and using a complex team of trained specialists. The principles of osteosynthesis in midface trauma respect the general principles of osteosynthesis. The prognosis depends on the associated pathology, age, social status, and correct assessment of viscerocranium lesions able to provide surgical and postop care. The current COVID-19 pandemic modifies the level of emergency care toward conservative attitude for trauma cases. Consider every trauma case as a possible COVID-19 suspect, and train the staff to equip quickly level 3 PPE. Keys to success are designing special access circuits for trauma cases reducing the time spent in the ER and subsequent referral of the case to specialized medical facilities treating COVID-19 cases.

Author details

Daniela Vrinceanu[1], Bogdan Banica[2] and Mihai Dumitru[1,3]*

1 ENT Department, Bucharest Emergency University Hospital, Bucharest, Romania

2 OMF Surgery Department, Bucharest Emergency University Hospital, Bucharest, Romania

3 Anatomy Department, Carol Davila University of Medicine and Pharmacy, Bucharest, Romania

*Address all correspondence to: orldumitrumihai@yahoo.com

References

[1] Scheyerer MJ, Döring R, Fuchs N, Metzler P, Sprengel K, Werner CML, et al. Maxillofacial injuries in severely injured patients. Journal of Trauma Management & Outcomes. 2015;**9**:4. DOI: 10.1186/s13032-015-0025-2

[2] Gadre KS, Halli R, Joshi S, Ramanojam S, Gadre PK, Kunchur R, et al. Incidence and pattern of cranio-maxillofacial injuries: A 22 year retrospective analysis of cases operated at major trauma hospitals/centres in Pune, India. Journal of Maxillofacial and Oral Surgery. 2013;**12**(4):372-378. DOI: 10.1007/s12663-012-0446-7

[3] Vrinceanu D, Banica B. Principles of surgical treatment in the midface trauma—Theory and practice. Maedica – a Journal of Clinical Medicine. 2014;**9**(4):361-366

[4] Sina C, Castoldi L, D'Orto O, Castaldi S. The value of protocols: The experience about a facial trauma protocol applied in the emergency room in a research and teaching hospital in the north part of Italy. Journal of Public Health Research. 2012;**1**(3):240-242. DOI: 10.4081/jphr.2012.e38

[5] Kraft A, Abermann E, Stigler R, Zsifkovits C, Pedross F, Kloss F, et al. Craniomaxillofacial trauma: Synopsis of 14,654 cases with 35,129 injuries in 15 years. Craniomaxillofacial Trauma & Reconstruction. 2012;**5**(1):41-50. DOI: 10.1055/s-0031-1293520

[6] Bajwa SJ, Kaur J, Singh A, Kapoor V, Bindra GS, Ghai GS. Clinical and critical care concerns of cranio-facial trauma: A retrospective study in a tertiary care institute. National Journal of Maxillofacial Surgery. 2012;**3**(2):133-138. DOI: 10.4103/0975-5950.111343

[7] Koryczan P, Zapała J, Wyszyńska-Pawelec G. Reduction in visual acuity and intraocular injuries in orbital floor fracture. Folia Medica Cracoviensia. 2015;**55**(3):49-56

[8] Mishra RK, Munivenkatappa A, Prathyusha V, Shukla DP, Devi BI. Clinical predictors of abnormal head computed tomography scan in patients who are conscious after head injury. Journal of Neuroscience in Rural Practice. 2017;**8**(1):64-67. DOI: 10.4103/0976-3147.193538

[9] Roman R, Hedeşiu M, Fildan F, Ileşan R, Mitea D, Dinu C, et al. The use of reformatted cone beam CT images in assessing mid-face trauma, with a focus on the orbital floor fractures. Clujul Medical. 2016;**89**(4):519-524

[10] Anghel I, Anghel AG, Soreanu CC, Dumitru M. Craniofacial trauma produced by a violent mechanism. Coltea ENT Clinic experience. Romanian Journal of Legal Medicine. 2012;**20**:215-218. DOI: 10.4323/rjlm.2012.215

[11] Roumeliotis G, Ahluwalia R, Jenkyn T, Yazdani A. The Le Fort system revisited: Trauma velocity predicts the path of Le Fort I fractures through the lateral buttress. Plastic Surgery (Oakv). 2015;**23**(1):40-42

[12] Chandra L, Deepa D, Atri M, Pandey SM, Passi D, Goyal J, et al. A retrospective cross-sectional study of maxillofacial trauma in Delhi-NCR region. Journal of Family Medicine and Primary Care. 2019;**8**(4):1453-1459. DOI: 10.4103/jfmpc.jfmpc_89_19

[13] Chin YP, Leno MB, Dumrongwongsiri S, Chung KH, Lin HH, Lo LJ. The pterygomaxillary junction: An imaging study for surgical information of LeFort I osteotomy. Scientific Reports. 2017;**7**(1):9953. DOI: 10.1038/s41598-017-10592-8

[14] Louis M, Agrawal N, Truong TA. Midface fractures II. Seminars in Plastic Surgery. 2017;**31**(2):94-99. DOI: 10.1055/s-0037-1601373

[15] Rajkumar GC, Ashwin DP, Singh R, Prashanth R, Rudresh KB. Ocular injuries associated with midface fractures: A 5 year survey. Journal of Maxillofacial and Oral Surgery. 2015;**14**(4):925-929. DOI: 10.1007/s12663-015-0778-1

[16] Menon S, Sham ME, Kumar V, Archana S, Nath P, Shivakotee S, et al. Maxillofacial fracture patterns in road traffic accidents. Annals of Maxillofacial Surgery. 2019;**9**(2):345-348. DOI: 10.4103/ams.ams_136_19

[17] Septa D, Newaskar VP, Agrawal D, Tibra S. Etiology, incidence and patterns of mid-face fractures and associated ocular injuries. Journal of Maxillofacial and Oral Surgery. 2014;**13**(2):115-119. DOI: 10.1007/s12663-012-0452-9

[18] Abiodun A, Atinuke A, Yvonne O. Computerized tomography assessment of cranial and mid-facial fractures in patients following road traffic accident in south-west Nigeria. Annals of African Medicine. 2012;**11**(3):131-138. DOI: 10.4103/1596-3519.96860

[19] Pappachan B, Alexander M. Biomechanics of cranio-maxillofacial trauma. Journal of Maxillofacial and Oral Surgery. 2012;**11**(2):224-230. DOI: 10.1007/s12663-011-0289-7

[20] Businger AP, Krebs J, Schaller B, Zimmermann H, Exadaktylos AK. Cranio-maxillofacial injuries in victims of interpersonal violence. Swiss Medical Weekly. 2012;**142**:w13687. DOI: 10.4414/smw.2012.13687

[21] Waterkamp V, Ricklin M, Schaller B, Katsoulis K, Exadaktylos A. Severity and pattern of injuries caused by the traditional Swiss team sport 'Hornussen': First retrospective study at a level I trauma centre in Switzerland. BMJ Open Sport & Exercise Medicine. 2016;**2**(1):e000122

[22] Ghabach MB, Abou Rouphael MA, Roumoulian CE, Helou MR. Airway management in a patient with Le Fort III fracture. Saudi Journal of Anaesthesia. 2014;**8**(1):128-130. DOI: 10.4103/1658-354X.125974

[23] Olayemi AB, Adeniyi AO, Samuel U, Emeka OA. Pattern, severity, and management of cranio-maxillofacial soft-tissue injuries in Port Harcourt, Nigeria. Journal of Emergencies, Trauma, and Shock. 2013;**6**(4):235-240. DOI: 10.4103/0974-2700.120362

[24] Vrinceanu D, Banica B, Dumitru M, Musat G. Advantages of the open approach in sinonasal tract tumors with midfacial and suprastructure invasion. R.j. of Rhinology. 2020;**10**(37):30-34. DOI: 10.2478/rjr-2020-0007

[25] Giran G, Paré A, Croisé B, Koudougou C, Mercier JM, Laure B, et al. Radiographic evaluation of percutaneous transfacial wiring versus open internal fixation for surgical treatment of unstable zygomatic bone fractures. PLoS One. 2019;**14**(8):e0220913. DOI: 10.1371/journal.pone.0220913

[26] Hartwig S, Nissen MC, Voss JO, Doll C, Adolphs N, Heiland M, et al. Clinical outcome after orbital floor fracture reduction with special regard to patient's satisfaction. Chinese Journal of Traumatology. 2019;**22**(3):155-160. DOI: 10.1016/j.cjtee.2019.01.002

[27] Nekooei S, Sardabi M, Razavi ME, Nekooei A, Kiarudi MY. Implantation of customized, preshaped implant for orbital fractures with the aid of three-dimensional printing. Middle East African Journal of Ophthalmology.

2018;**25**(1):56-58. DOI: 10.4103/meajo.MEAJO_262_16

[28] Han DG. Considerations for nasal bone fractures: Preoperative, perioperative, and postoperative. Archives of Craniofacial Surgery. 2020;**21**(1):3-6. DOI: 10.7181/acfs.2020.00031

[29] Kang BH, Kang HS, Han JJ, Jung S, Park HJ, Oh HK, et al. A retrospective clinical investigation for the effectiveness of closed reduction on nasal bone fracture. Maxillofacial Plastic and Reconstructive Surgery. 2019;**41**(1):53. DOI: 10.1186/s40902-019-0236-y

[30] Onişor-Gligor F, Ţenţ PA, Bran S, Juncar M. A naso-orbito-ethmoid (NOE) fracture associated with bilateral anterior and posterior frontal sinus wall fractures caused by a horse kick-case report and short literature review. Medicina (Kaunas, Lithuania). 2019;**55**(11). pii: E731. DOI: 10.3390/medicina55110731

[31] Park CH, Chung KJ, Kim TG, Lee JH, Kim IK, Kim YH. Big data statistical analysis of facial fractures in Korea. Journal of Korean Medical Science. 2020;**35**(7):e57. DOI: 10.3346/jkms.2020.35.e57

[32] Teng TS, Ishak NL, Subha ST, Bakar SA. Traumatic transnasal penetrating injury with cerebral spinal fluid leak. EXCLI Journal. 2019;**18**:223-228. DOI: 10.17179/excli2018-1971

[33] Mourad M, Inman JC, Chan DM, Ducic Y. Contemporary trends in the management of posttraumatic cerebrospinal fluid leaks. Craniomaxillofacial Trauma & Reconstruction. 2018;**11**(1):71-77. DOI: 10.1055/s-0036-1584890

[34] Hasheminia D, Kalantar Motamedi MR, Hashemzehi H, Nazeri R, Movahedian B. A 7-year study of 1,278 patients with maxillofacial trauma and cerebrospinal fluid leak. Journal of Maxillofacial and Oral Surgery. 2015;**14**(2):258-262. DOI: 10.1007/s12663-014-0630-z

[35] Lee EI, Mohan K, Koshy JC, Hollier LH Jr. Optimizing the surgical management of zygomaticomaxillary complex fractures. Seminars in Plastic Surgery. 2010;**24**(4):389-397. DOI: 10.1055/s-0030-1269768

[36] Borrelli MR, Hu MS, Longaker MT, Lorenz HP. Tissue engineering and regenerative medicine in craniofacial reconstruction and facial aesthetics. The Journal of Craniofacial Surgery. 2020;**31**(1):15-27. DOI: 10.1097/SCS.0000000000005840

[37] Olsson P, Nysjö F, Hirsch JM, Carlbom IB. A haptics-assisted cranio-maxillofacial surgery planning system for restoring skeletal anatomy in complex trauma cases. International Journal of Computer Assisted Radiology and Surgery. 2013;**8**(6):887-894. DOI: 10.1007/s11548-013-0827-5

[38] Sharma S, Nanda A, Koli D, Daksh S, Verma M. Role of a dentist in comprehensive management of a comatose patient with post traumatic head injury and neuropathological chewing. Indian Journal of Palliative Care. 2014;**20**(2):146-152. DOI: 10.4103/0973-1075.132639

[39] Mottini M, Wolf R, Soong PL, Lieger O, Nakahara K, Schaller B. The role of postoperative antibiotics in facial fractures: Comparing the efficacy of a 1-day versus a prolonged regimen. Journal of Trauma and Acute Care Surgery. 2014;**76**(3):720-724. DOI: 10.1097/TA.0000000000000123

[40] Campos GB, Lucena EE, da Silva JS, Gomes PP, Germano AR. Efficacy assessment of two antibiotic prophylaxis regimens in oral and maxillofacial

trauma surgery: Preliminary results. International Journal of Clinical and Experimental Medicine. 2015;**8**(2):2846-2852

[41] Ikeda K, Sakurada T, Takasaka T, Okitsu T, Yoshida S. Anosmia following head trauma: Preliminary study of steroid treatment. The Tohoku Journal of Experimental Medicine. 1995;**177**(4):343-351

[42] Vrinceanu D, Dumitru M, Banica B, Nica A. Foreign body in maxillary sinus with skin fistula. Journal of Surgical Sciences. 2019;**6**(3):82-84. DOI: 10.33695/jss.v6i3.278

[43] Alwani M, Jones AJ, Sandelski M, Bandali E, Lancaster B, Sim MW, et al. Facing facts: Facial injuries from stand-up electric scooters. Cureus. 2020;**12**(1):e6663. DOI: 10.7759/cureus.6663

[44] Breeze J, Bowley DM, Combes JG, Baden J, Rickard RF, DuBose J, et al. Facial injury management undertaken at US and UK medical treatment facilities during the Iraq and Afghanistan conflicts: A retrospective cohort study. BMJ Open. 2019;**9**(11):e033557. DOI: 10.1136/bmjopen-2019-033557

[45] Choi DS, Lee JW, Yang JD, Chung HY, Cho BC, Choi KY. Minimal packing duration in close reduction for nasal bone fracture treatment. Journal of Plastic Surgery and Hand Surgery. 2015;**49**(5):275-279. DOI: 10.3109/2000656X.2015.1034726

[46] Koh JH, Bhatti O, Mahmood A, Agar N. Traumatic nasal injuries in general practice. Australian Family Physician. 2016;**45**(9):650-653

[47] Ehmedah A, Nedeljkovic P, Dacic S, Repac J, Draskovic Pavlovic B, Vucevic D, et al. Vitamin B complex treatment attenuates local inflammation after peripheral nerve injury. Molecules. 2019;**24**(24). pii: E4615. DOI: 10.3390/molecules24244615

[48] Pullar JM, Carr AC, Vissers MCM. The roles of vitamin C in skin health. Nutrients. 2017;**9**(8). pii: E866. DOI: 10.3390/nu9080866

[49] Wilson N, Heke S, Holmes S, Dain V, Priebe S, Bridle C, et al. Prevalence and predictive factors of psychological morbidity following facial injury: A prospective study of patients attending a maxillofacial outpatient clinic within a major UK city. Dialogues in Clinical Neuroscience. 2018;**20**(4):327-339

[50] Zeiderman MR, Pu LLQ. Contemporary reconstruction after complex facial trauma. Burns Trauma. 2020;**8**:tkaa003. DOI: 10.1093/burnst/tkaa003

[51] Gómez Roselló E, Quiles Granado AM, Artajona Garcia M, Juanpere Martí S, Laguillo Sala G, Beltrán Mármol B, et al. Facial fractures: Classification and highlights for a useful report. Insights Into Imaging. 2020;**11**(1):49. DOI: 10.1186/s13244-020-00847-w

[52] Liu FC, Halsey JN, Oleck NC, Lee ES, Granick MS. Facial fractures as a result of falls in the elderly: Concomitant injuries and management strategies. Craniomaxillofacial Trauma & Reconstruction. 2019;**12**(1):45-53. DOI: 10.1055/s-0038-1642034

[53] Coccolini F, Perrone G, Chiarugi M, Di Marzo F, Ansaloni L, Scandroglio I, et al. Surgery in COVID-19 patients: Operational directives. World Journal of Emergency Surgery. 2020;**15**(1):25. DOI: 10.1186/s13017-020-00307-2

[54] Livingston DH, Bonne S, Morello C, Fox A. Optimizing the trauma resuscitation bay during the covid-19 pandemic. Trauma Surgery &

Acute Care Open. 2020;**5**(1):e000488. DOI: 10.1136/tsaco-2020-000488

[55] Gok AFK, Eryılmaz M, Ozmen MM, Alimoglu O, Ertekin C, Kurtoglu MH. Recommendations for trauma and emergency general surgery practice during COVID-19 pandemic. Ulusal Travma ve Acil Cerrahi Dergisi. 2020;**26**(3):335-342. DOI: 10.14744/tjtes.2020.79954

Chapter 7

Designing Flaps for Closure of a Variety of Skin Defects

Alfredo Alvarado

Abstract

In this article, I am presenting a variety of working models for closure of skin defects of different shapes along with their corresponding indications and mode of use. These working models can be enlarged or reduced in size using a regular copying machine in order to evaluate the best possibilities related to the position of the incision. The great advantage of this method is that the geometric results are always predictable. Furthermore, this method will improve the survival of the flaps and the cosmetic results. In summary, the surgeon can use a variety of skin incisions taking advantage of the minimal tension lines of the skin and also taking into consideration the anatomical characteristics of the region involved. In this article, I have used the minimal tension lines of the skin, because they are easy to demonstrate by simple measures, such as pinching of the skin in different directions. In addition, the surgeon can assess the mobility and the elasticity of the skin on an individual basis.

Keywords: skin defects closure, soft tissue flaps, pedicled skin flaps, reciprocal incisions, circular and semicircular incisions, triangular incisions, oval and elongated hexagonal incisions, skin minimal tension lines, relaxed skin tension lines

1. Introduction

When excising large skin lesions, the ideal incision is a circular one, since most of the skin lesions are round, and because it provides an adequate margin of resection, and at the same time will avoid the removal of sound skin. The main problem with this approach is that the resultant circular defect may prove to be very difficult to close. To solve this problem, the surgeon can use different incisions that can be closed in a more expedite way and with better cosmetic results. Another alternative would be a split-thickness skin graft, which sometimes would not match the color or texture of the recipient area [1–3].

It is for these reasons that the surgeon has to use different methods such as using a rhombic or elliptical incision that leaves a long suture line and will waste more sound skin. In some cases, the circular incision can be transformed into a square incision, such as the Dufourmentel flap [4], or into a rhomboid defect, such as the Limberg flap [5], but both of them will generate loss of sound skin. The Limberg method for closure of a hexagonal defect uses three triangular flaps, but these flaps are rather small which may compromise their survival. Besides this, the resultant triangular suture line is not cosmetically acceptable.

 IntechOpen

2. Closure of circular skin defects

I designed three "reciprocal incisions" in 1981 aiming to close large circular defects [6] with minimal waste of sound skin and at the same time to avoid the formation of dog ears. The first one is the *double S incision* (**Figure 1**) that is adequate for small defects in which the skin is fairly elastic. The second one is the *bow tie incision* (**Figure 2**) that is indicated in intermediate defects in which the skin is quite elastic. The third incision is the *combined V incision* (**Figure 3**) that is valuable for large defects in which the skin is fairly elastic. These incisions should be considered in view of the anatomical characteristics of the skin, such as the natural creases or the minimal tension lines. In certain cases, the surgeon quite often encounters a problem when the lesion is located in a confined anatomical area or when the

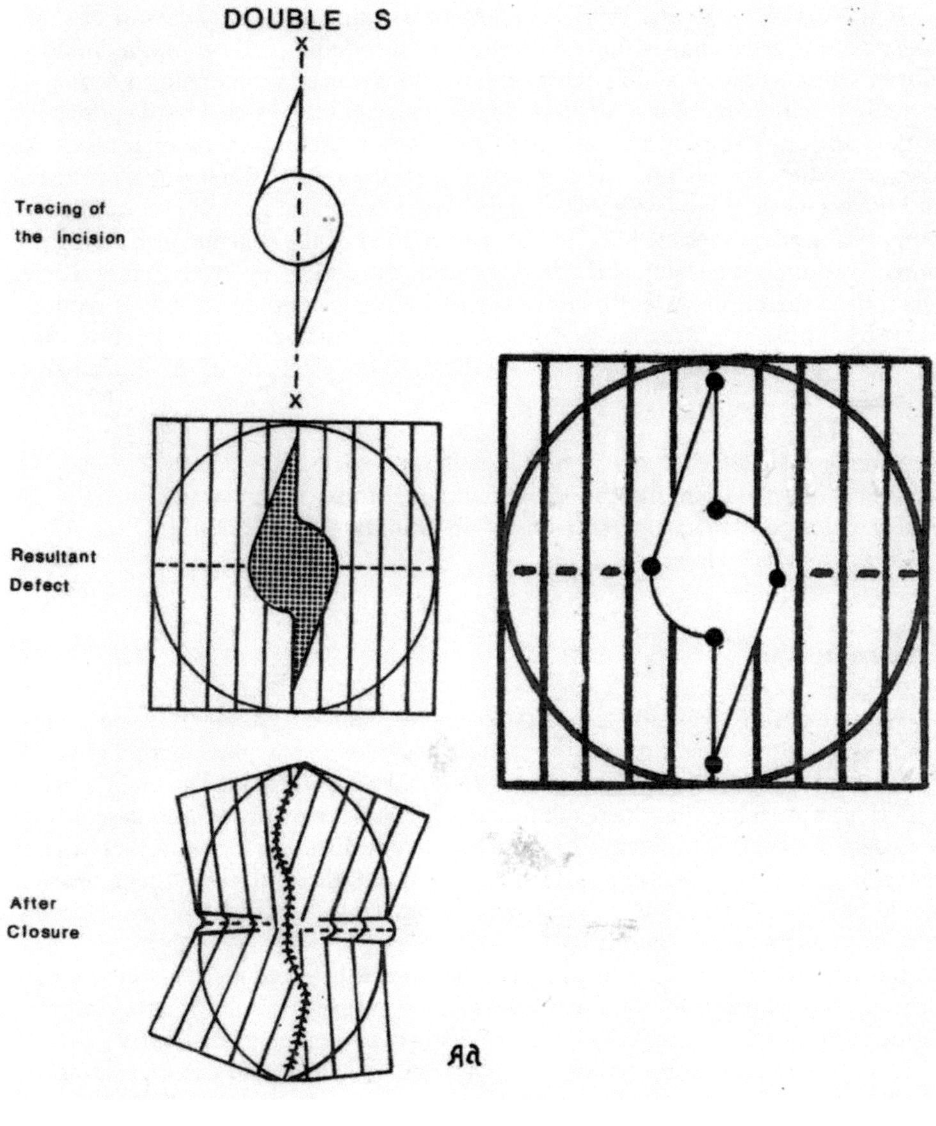

Figure 1.
Here, the double S incision represents half of the rhombic incision which has a wastage of 103%, so the wastage of skin is reduced in half and the resultant suture line shows a mild wave shape. The vertical lines represent the minimal tension lines of the skin, and the axis X-X represents the center of these lines.

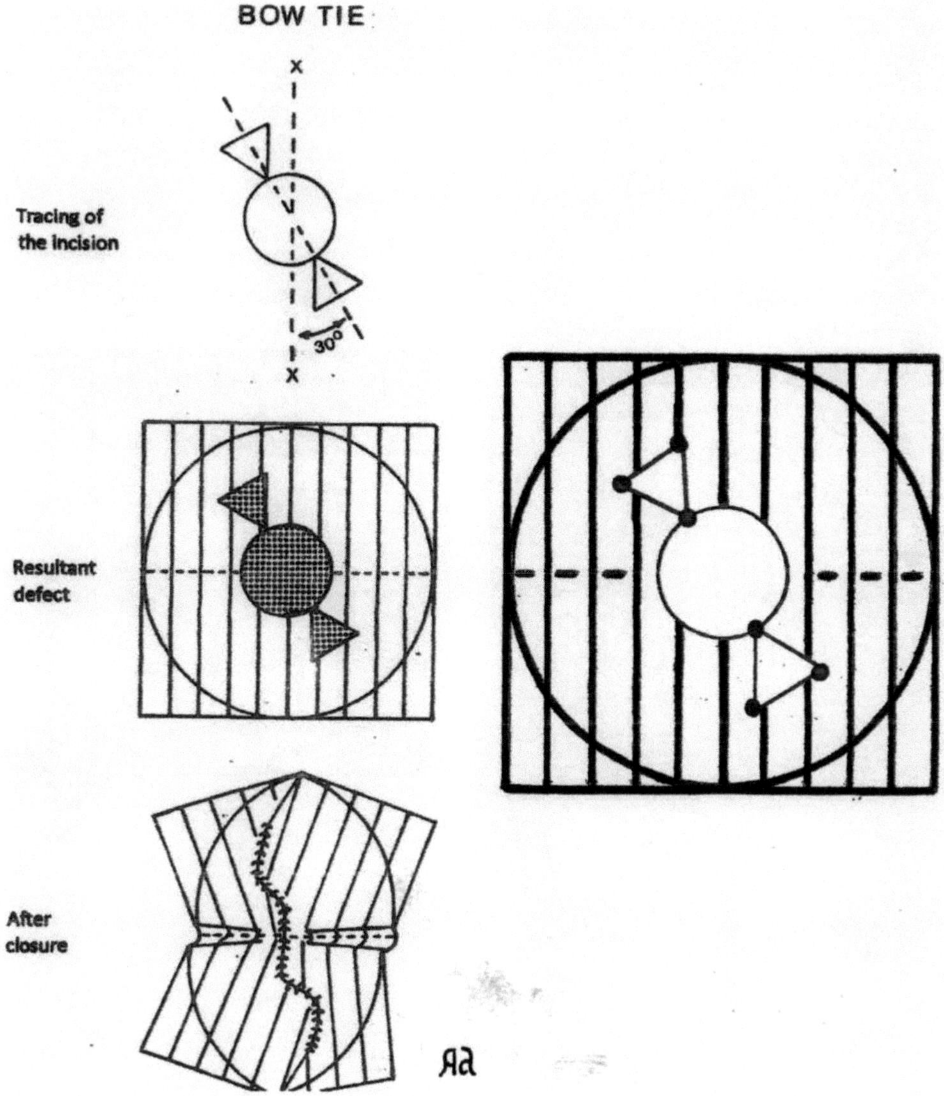

Figure 2.
The bow tie incision is one of the reciprocal incisions in which the length of both sides of the incision is equal, which eliminates the formation of dog ears. The wastage of sound skin for this incision is 36%.

elasticity of the skin is limited or when the lesion is too large. To obviate these problems, I published various methods for closure of circular and semicircular skin defects in 2016 [7, 8].

For circular skin defects, two incisions were described, the *cat's ear* (**Figure 4**) and the *bird's beak* (**Figure 5**) incisions that are very versatile because they can adapt to different anatomic configurations. The first one is a modification of the *bow tie* incision and the second one is a modification of the *combined V* incision mentioned before. They require minimal dissection of the flaps and produce a relative short suture line. The cat's ear and the bird beak's incisions have the great advantage of allowing the positioning of the incision along the normal creases of the skin which will produce better cosmetic results. For instance, the bird's beak incision is very useful when dealing with a skin lesion near the eye [5] or when dealing with a pilonidal cyst that is too low and near the anus.

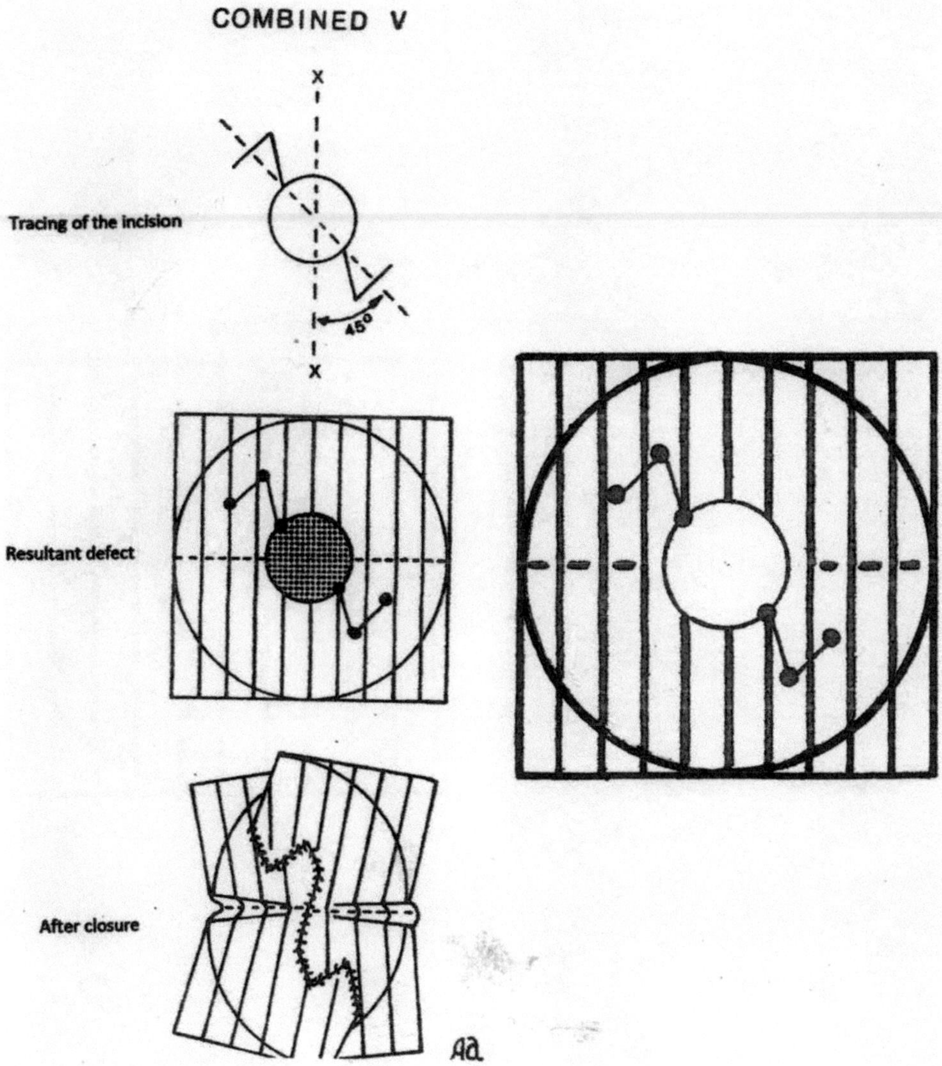

Figure 3.
The combined V incision is other reciprocal incision that is very useful when trying to save sound skin, since the wastage of the skin is reduced to 0%. It could be very useful for removal of large skin lesions because the wastage of sound skin is null.

3. Closure of semicircular skin defects

For semicircular skin defects, two incisions were described, the *half-moon* (**Figure 6**) and the *goblet* (**Figure 7**) incisions. The first one was especially designed for closure of semicircular defects, and the second one for closure of robust semicircular defects. Both incisions do not have a basic extension but have a complementary extension at the curved side of the incision. The axis of the incisions (axis X-X) follows the minimal tension lines and is centered at the upper corner of the incision. The calculated wastage for the cat's ear incision is 41 and 24% for the bird's beak incision which is in contrast to the wastage of 21% for the half-moon incision and 19% for the goblet incision. All of these configurations are much better as compared with the ellipsoid incision that has a wastage of 156% [6]. One advantage of the goblet incision is that it is more versatile because it has two options for the rotation of the flaps.

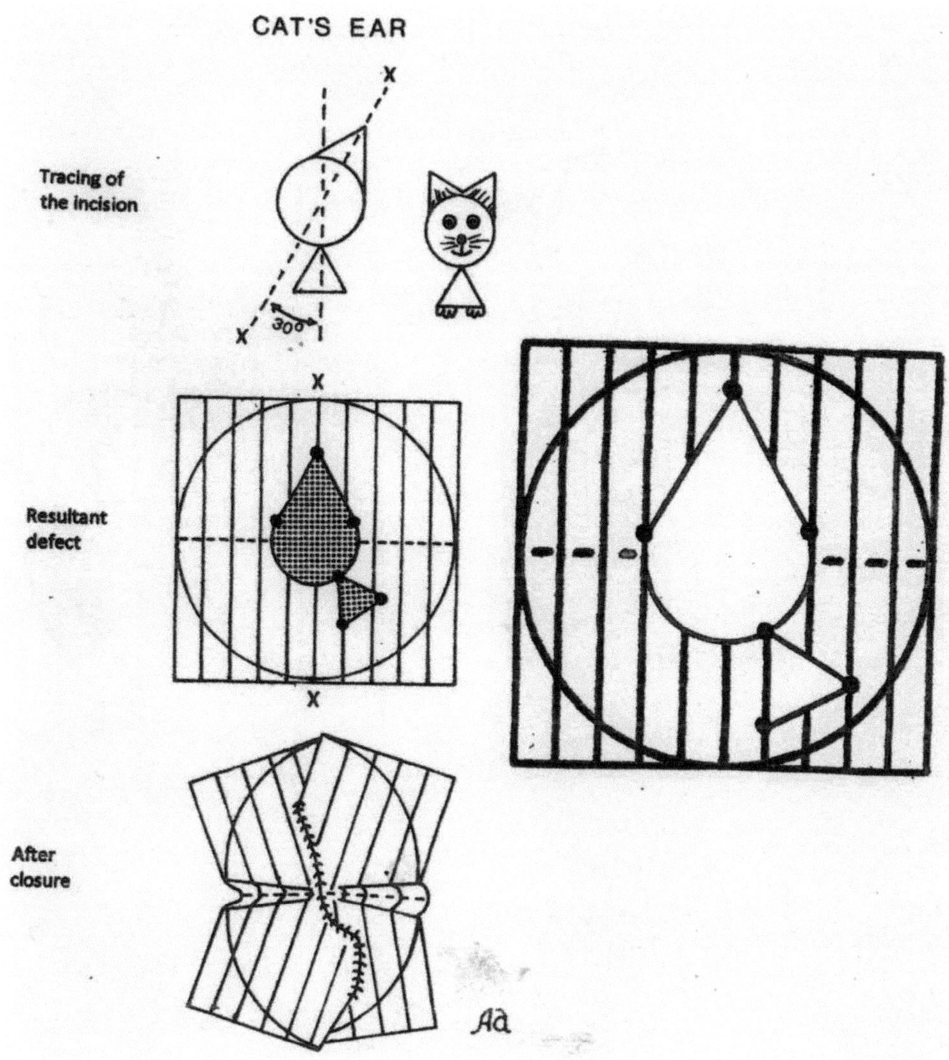

Figure 4.
The cat's ear incision is very useful for skin lesions of the face, where the suture line has to follow the minimal tension lines of the skin. The wastage of skin for this incision is 41%.

4. Closure of triangular skin defects

Most of times, skin lesions have a round shape; but in certain cases, the lesions could present themselves in a triangular shape. In the recent medical literature, there are few methods that can be used for closure of triangular skin defects such as the L-shaped flap for triangular skin defects of Sakai and Soeda [9] and the Mutaf triangular closure [10], or the triangular excision for small lesions of Filho and colleagues [11]. The tracing of the first two incisions is rather complicated and the resultant flaps have a narrow base that could jeopardize their survival.

It is for these reasons that I published a "Simple method for closure of triangular skin defects" [12] in 2016. These incisions are easy to trace and to memorize, and more important, they are provided with wide base flaps. Furthermore, the resultant suture lines are away from the central area of the incision and the edges of the

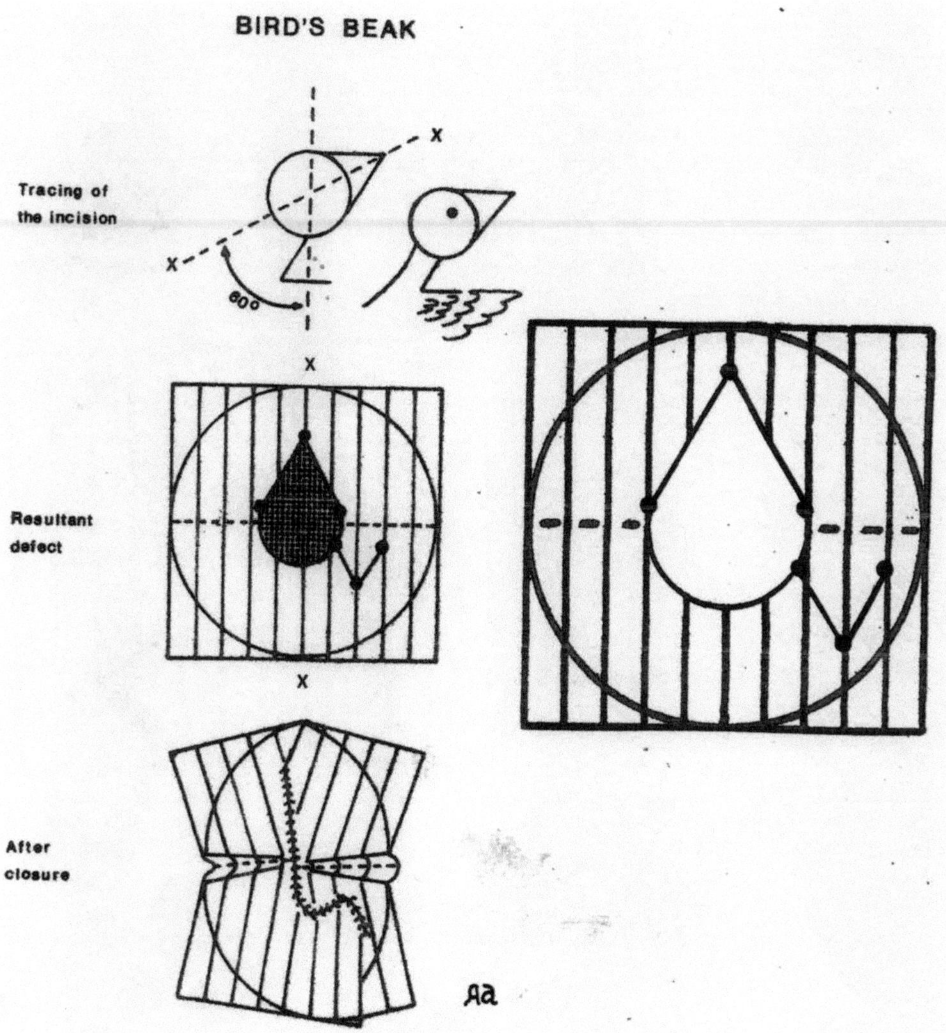

Figure 5.
The bird's beak incision is very useful in confined regions, where it is important to save sound skin as much as possible, for instance when dealing with lesions near to the orbit or nose. The wastage for this incision is 24%.

suture lines complies with the principle of reciprocity by which the edges of the skin end up even and without the formation of dog ears. In addition, these incisions have the advantage of producing a short suture line, as compared with the Sakai Soeda and the Mutaf incisions.

As a consequence, this simple method for closure of triangular skin defects could very useful for closure of large meningoceles or when resecting pilonidal sinuses or when removing triangular defects of the face. In the present article, these incisions have been slightly modified in order to produce a better suture line (**Figures 8** and **9**). Besides this, their tracing is easier to memorize, since the base of the triangles are always divided in half instead of dividing in quarters.

5. Closure of oval and elongated hexagonal skin defects

In some occasions, the skin defects take the configuration of an oval (**Figure 10**) or an elongated hexagon (**Figure 11**) which would require considerable extensions at their extremities that in some confined anatomical regions is not feasible.

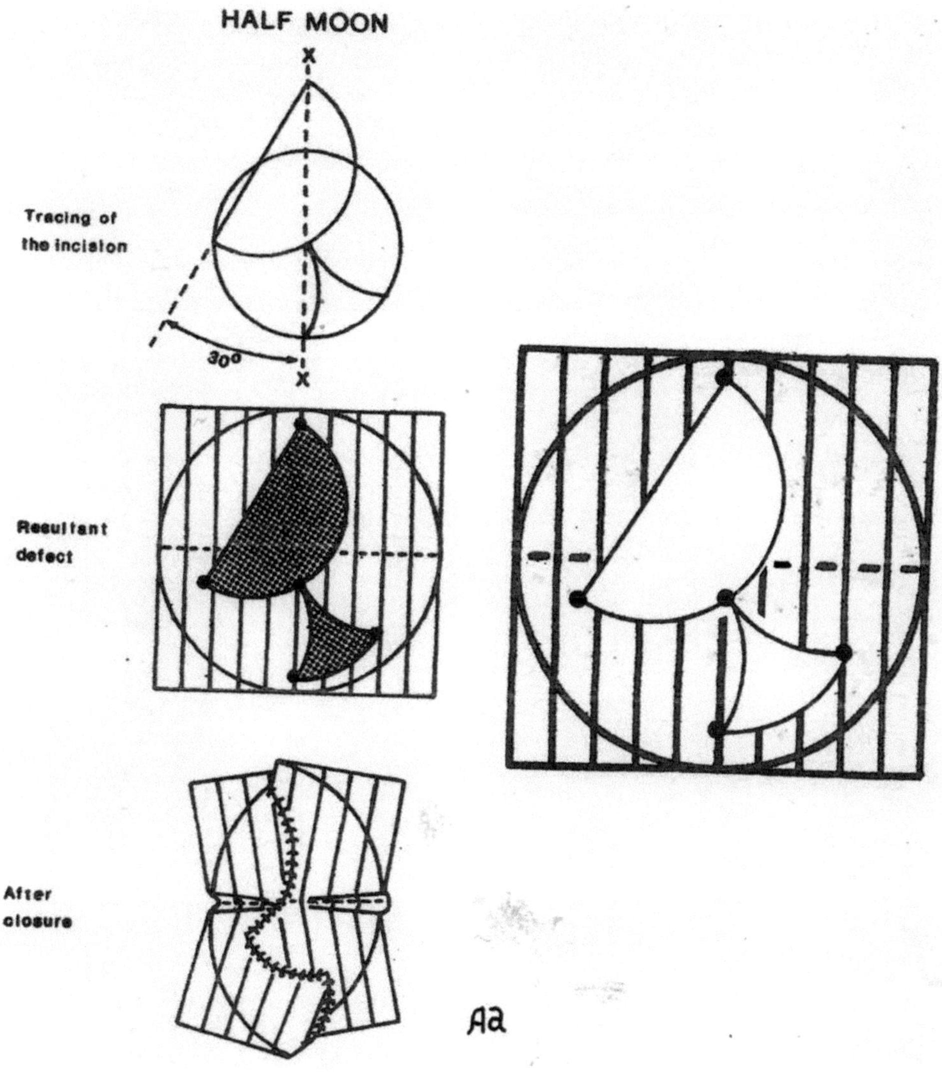

Figure 6.
The half-moon incision can be used for skin lesions of similar shape and have the advantage of saving sound skin. The wastage for this incision is 21%.

To solve this problem, I am presenting here two new paper models that are easy to trace and to memorize with the advantage of generating a short suture line and with practically no wastage of skin.

6. Indications

Any of the incisions described in this article can be selected to accommodate to the characteristics of a particular anatomical region. For instance, the **double S incision** (**Figure 1**) is indicated for closure of multiple small skin defects of the face and other parts of the body. This incision is useful in small defects of the scalp (>1 cm in diameter) and moderate defects of the face (2–3 cm in diameter).

The **bow tie incision** (**Figure 2**) is very useful when the skin is not quite elastic, such as in small defects of the scalp (1–2 cm in diameter), because the waste of sound skin for this incision is 36% only. For the same season, it is very useful in very large lesions of the trunk (5–10 cm in diameter).

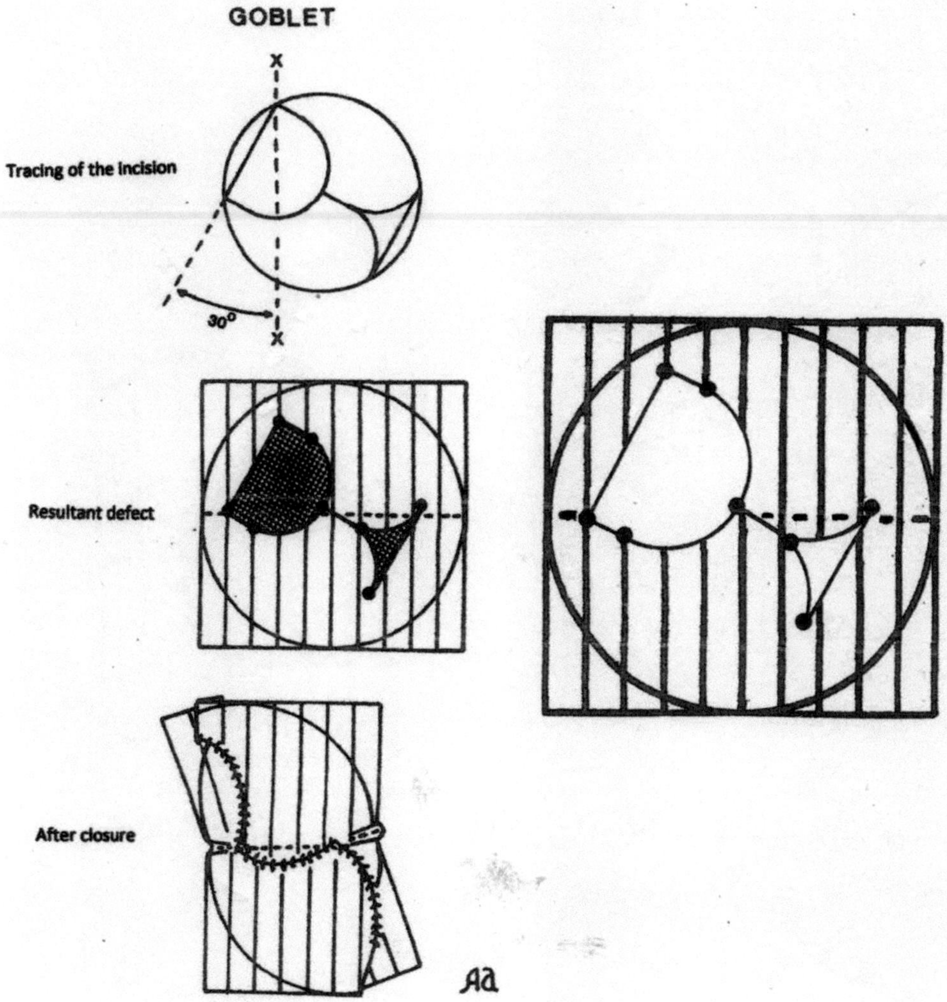

Figure 7.
The goblet incision is similar to the half-moon incision, but is more robust and saves more sound skin (19%).

The **combined V incision (Figure 3)** is indicated in very large defects of the scalp (more than 2 cm in diameter) because with this incision there is no wastage of normal skin. For the same reason, it is very useful in very large lesions of the thorax and abdomen where saving of sound skin is important.

The **cat's ear** and the **bird's beak incisions (Figures 4** and 5) are very convenient for closure of large lesions of the face near the eye and nose where the elasticity of the skin is poor and where a good cosmetic result is desired. These two incisions can be aligned following the natural creases of the skin so there is no distortion of the periorbital area or nose.

The **cat's ear** incision would be very useful in closing the skin defect after a radical mastectomy to prevent the formation of a large dog ear at the dorsal end of the incision. In this situation, the ear portion should point to the sternum and the complementary extension, below the axilla, eliminates the extension of the elliptical incision toward the back.

The **bird's beak incision** is very useful when dealing with a pilonidal cyst that is too low and near the anus. In this case, the beak should point upward and to the midline and the additional incision can be placed on either side at the lower side of the defect.

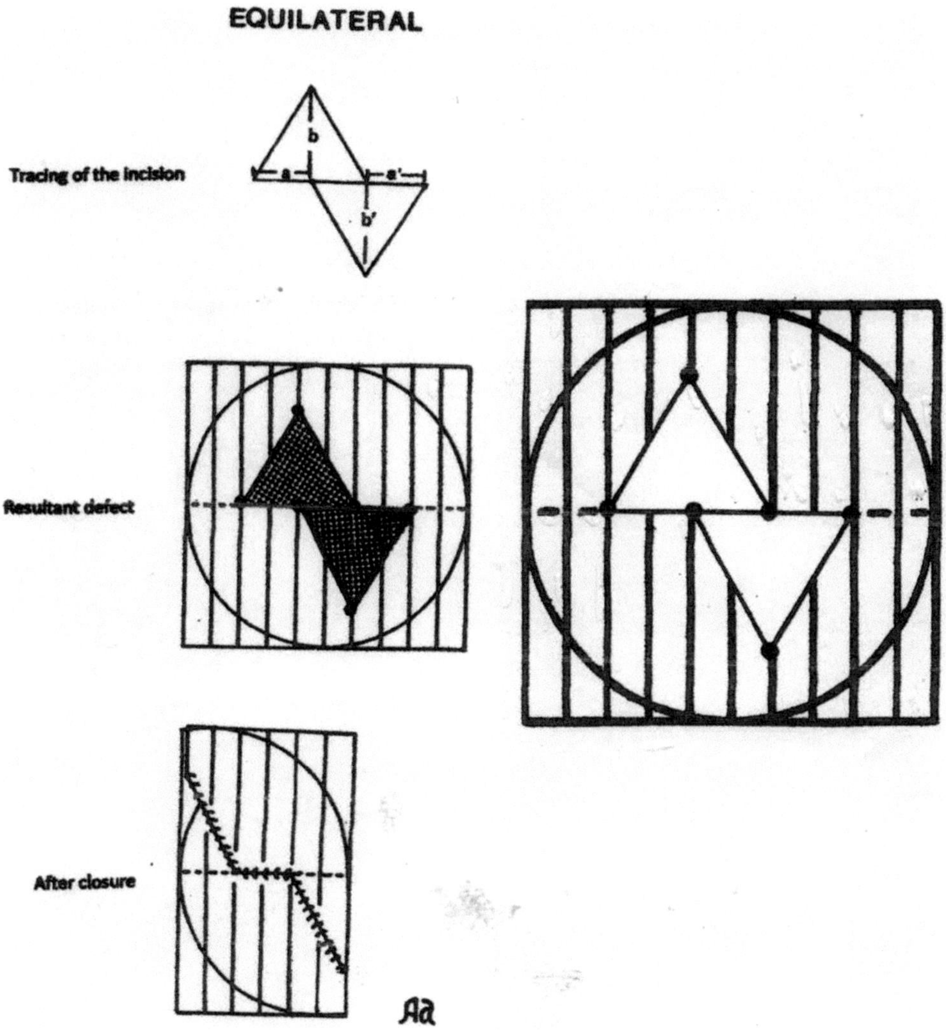

Figure 8.
The equilateral triangular incision is useful for lesions of similar shape, for instance when repairing meningoceles or when resecting pilonidal sinuses or when removing triangular defects of the infraorbital region. However, the wastage of sound skin for this incision is 100%, but this is better than the wastage of the rhomboid or elliptical incisions (103% and 156%, respectively).

The **half-moon** and the **goblet** incisions (**Figures 6** and 7) are indicated when the lesions have the same shape and when the surrounding skin is very scarce such as in the case of large meningoceles because the wastage of sound skin is minimal (29 and 19%, respectively). They are also indicated when dealing with large pressure ulcers of the sacral area or when dealing with pilonidal cysts where the defect should be closed with wide base flaps that should cover the skin defects avoiding a suture line in the middle of the defect.

The **triangular incisions** (**Figures 8** and **9**) are indicated when the skin lesions have a similar shape, and when the skin defect has to be covered with a suture line away from the central portion of the defect, such as in the case of large meningoceles. In these cases, the skin can be mobilized without compromising their blood supply since these incisions are provided with wide based flaps. These triangular incisions are also useful when resecting pilonidal sinuses or when removing triangular defects of the infraorbital region.

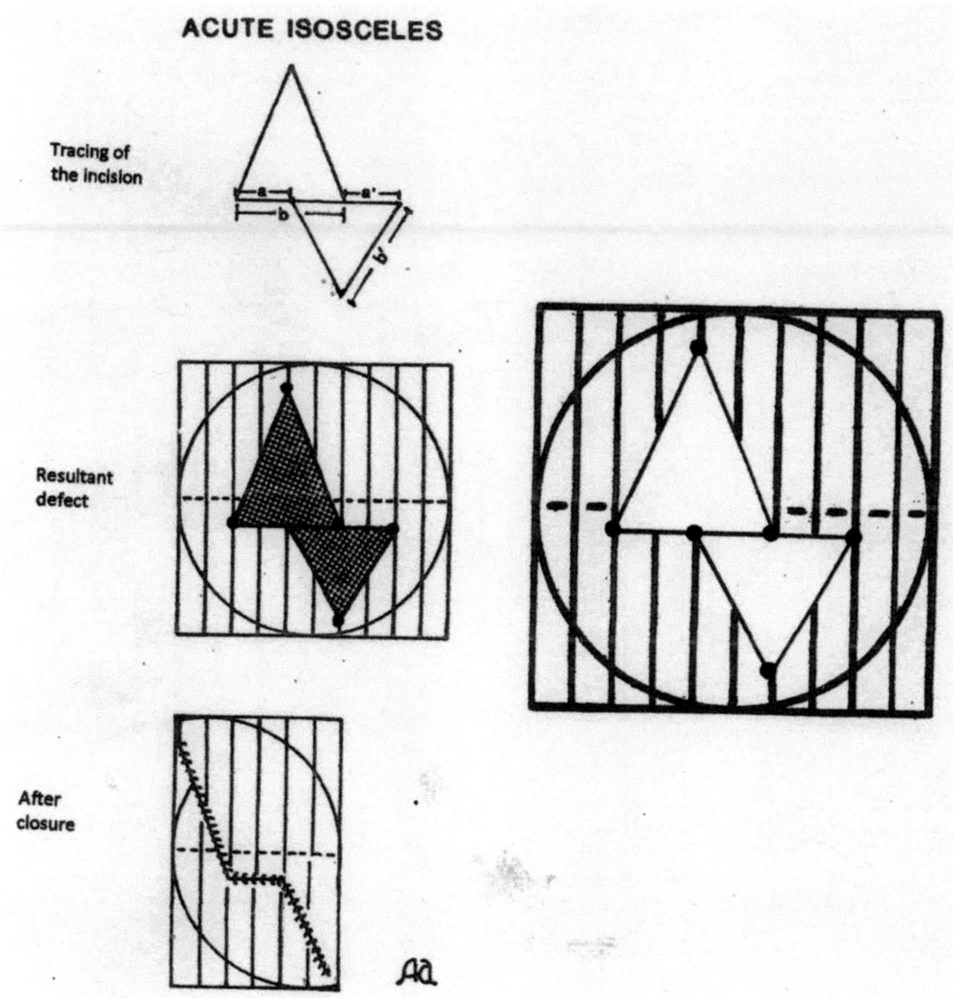

Figure 9.
The isosceles triangular incision is useful when excising lesions of similar shape, for instance pilonidal cysts or pressure ulcers of the sacral area. The wastage of sound skin is 71.4%.

The **oval** and the **elongated hexagonal** (**Figures 10** and **11**) incisions are indicated when the skin lesions have a similar shape and when there is not enough room for extension of the incision at the ends. Besides this, the wastage of normal skin for both incisions is essentially null.

7. Mode of use

For practical purposes, a working model of bond paper can be made to evaluate the different possibilities according to the anatomy and the particular conditions of the skin surrounding the lesion. The working models included here can be enlarged or reduced in size by using a regular copying machine, in advance of the operation. They could be used on the spot to test the more convenient position according to the size of the lesion to be removed. The center portion of the selected model can be removed in order to estimate the resection margins and the proper orientation of the incision.

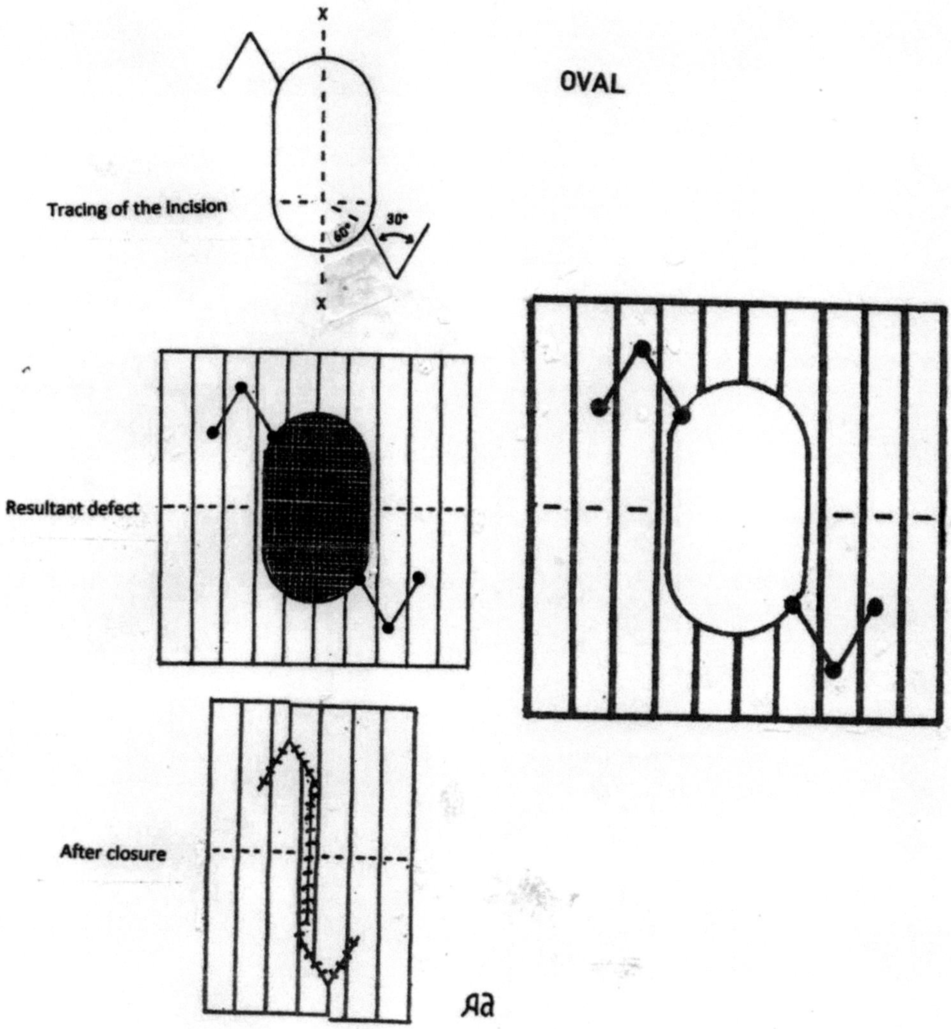

Figure 10.
The oval incision can be used for skin lesions of similar shape, for instance for two continuous round lesions. This incision would be very useful when removing large skin lesions of similar shape because the wastage of sound skin is null.

8. Summary

In this article, I am presenting a variety of working models for closure of skin defects of different shapes along with their corresponding indications and mode of use. These working models can be enlarged or reduced in size using a regular copying machine in order to evaluate the best possibilities related to the position of the incision. The great advantage of this method is that the geometrical results are always predictable. Furthermore, this method will improve the survival of the flaps and the cosmetic results.

9. Conclusion

In summary, the surgeon can use a variety of skin incisions taking advantage of the minimal tension lines of the skin and also taking into consideration the

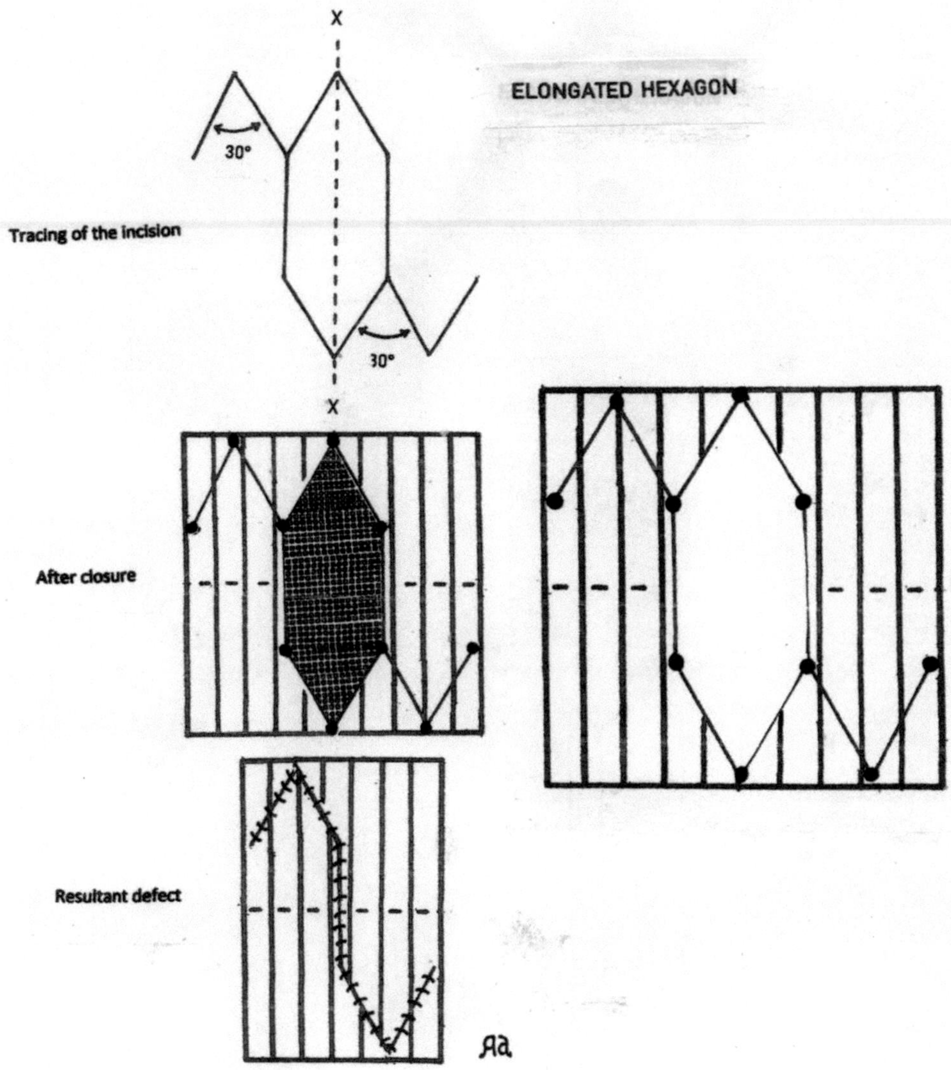

Figure 11.
The elongated hexagonal incision is easy to trace and to memorize because it is constructed by using straight lines only. This incision is useful when there is not enough room for extension of the incision at the ends, such as in the case of large skin lesions or sacral ulcers. The skin wastage for this incision is practically null.

anatomical characteristics of the region involved. For this purpose, the paper models described here can be prepared in advance of the planed surgery to make sure that they adapt to a particular location and according to the elasticity and mobility of the surrounding skin.

Author details

Alfredo Alvarado[1,2,3,4,5]

1 Universidad Nacional de Colombia, Bogotá, Colombia

2 American Board of Surgery and the American Board of Emergency Medicine, Miami, FL, USA

3 International College of Surgery, Chicago, IL, USA

4 Society of Laparoscopic Surgeons, Chicago, IL, USA

5 American College of Emergency Physicians, Irving, TX, USA

*Address all correspondence to: alfredoalvara@hotmail.com

References

[1] Paul SP. Biodynamic excisional skin tension (BEST) lines: Revisiting Langer's lines, skin biomechanics, current concepts in cutaneous surgery, and the (lack of) science behind skin lines used for surgical excisions. Journal of Dermatological Research. 2017;**2**(1):77-87

[2] Wilhelm BJ, Blackwell SJ, Phillips LG. Langer's lines: To use or not to use. Plastic and Reconstructive Surgery. 1999;**104**(1):205-214

[3] Lemperle G, Tenemhaus M, Knapp D, Lemperle SM. The direction of optimal skin incisions derived from striae distensae. Plastic and Reconstructive Surgery. 2014;**13**(6):1424-1434

[4] Dufourmentel C, Talaat SM. The kite-flap. In: Transactions of the Fifth International Congress of Plastic and Reconstructive Surgery. Melbourne: Butterworth; 1971. p. 1223

[5] Limberg AA. The Planning of Local Plastic Operations on the Body Surface. Theory and Practice. Lexington: Collamore; 1984

[6] Alvarado A. Reciprocal incisions for closure of circular skin defects. Plastic and Reconstructive Surgery. 1981;**67**:482-491

[7] Alvarado A. Designing flaps for closure of circular and semicircular skin defects. Plastic and Reconstructive Surgery. Global Open. 2015. DOI: 10.1097/GOX.0000000000000583; Published on Line

[8] Alvarado A. Three surgical cases about the use of pedicled flaps for closure of circular and semicircular skin defects. Plastic Surgery and Modern Techniques. 2019;**6**:145. DOI: 10.29011/2577-100045

[9] Sakai S, Soeda S. L-shaped flap for triangular slin defects. British Journal of Plastic Surgery. 1988;**41**:628-632

[10] Mutaf M, Bekericiouglu M, Erkulu I, Bulut O. A new technique for closure of large meningocele defects. Annals of Plastic Surgery. 2007;**59**:538-543

[11] Filho EA, Wojcik L, Brenner FA, Santamaria JR, Werner B. Cutaneous triangular excision with primary closure. Surgical and Cosmetic Dermatology. 2011;**3**:31-35

[12] Alvarado A. A simple method for closure of triangular skin defects. Advances in Plastic & Reconstructive Surgery. 2017;**1**(1):100-107

Chapter 8

Finesse in Damage Control Reconstruction for Trauma in Plastic Surgery

Shihheng Chen, Hung-Chi Chen and Yueh-Bih Tang

Abstract

Reconstructions of body, extremity and facial resurfacing facial defects are common encounters in plastic surgery. It may be owing to trauma, burn injury, tumor, congenital anomalies, miscellaneous kinds of malignancies. The face has its specific landmarks: the forehead, eyebrows, eyes with upper and lower eyelids, orbit, midface (nose, maxilla, zygoma), upper lip, cheeks, nasolabial folds, lower face (lower lip, mandible with angle), oral mucosa (buccal mucosa, upper lip sulcus, lower lip sulcus), mentum, and neck. Anatomical landmarks include forehead, eyebrow, and eyelids: upper/lower, orbit, midface: nose, maxilla, upper lip, nasolabial folds, and zygoma. Lower face: lower lip, mandible, oral mucosa, buccal mucosa, upper lip sulcus, lower lip sulcus. Strategic approaches include the following: tissue expansion, resection of tumor, and repair with resurfacing, repair of multilayer defect repair for functional purpose. Reconstruction for trauma is commonly encountered in the daily practice in plastic surgery. The trauma may be caused by miscellaneous causes, including traffic accident, fall, cutting, avulsion, contusion, electrical injuries, irradiation injuries, chemical injuries, etc., resulting in disfigurement, deformity and functional disabilities. The strategic approach is to achieve anatomical restoration, functional rehabilitation and aesthetic refinements for the afflicted individuals. Pursuing excellence in plastic surgery, bringing excellence to life is always the ultimate goal for plastic surgeons.

Keywords: reconstruction, anatomical restoration, functional rehabilitation, strategic approaches, aesthetic refinements

1. Introduction (Plastic surgery)

1.1 Anatomical restoration functional rehabilitation, aesthetic refinement are main goals in plastic surgery

The aim of plastic surgery is to achieve anatomical restoration, functional rehabilitation, aesthetic refinements.

1.1.1 Functional reconstruction for trauma

Post-trauma functional reconstruction involves solving scar contractures, restoration of nerve function, tendon or muscle function or body integrity.

1.1.2 Extremity reconstruction for trauma

Trauma to the extremities include partial or complete severance of body parts, injuries to major artery, vein, or nerve or tendon, all may cause different degree of functional disabilities and possible disfigurement.

1.1.3 Aesthetic facial reconstruction for trauma

Trauma at face with tissue defects are common encounters [1]. It may be caused by laceration, avulsion, contusion, burn injury, electrical injury, tumor, congenital anomalies [2–4], infections [5], miscellaneous kinds of malignancies and related treatments [6–9], radiation necrosis [10–11], etc.

1.1.4 Demarcation

The face has its specific landmarks [8]: the forehead, eyebrows, eyes with upper and lower eyelids, nose, upper and lower lips, cheeks, nasolabial folds, mandible with angles and mentum, and neck. Dynamic facial expressions and chewing, mastication are specific functions of face.

2. Strategic approaches

Strategic approaches should follow the demarcation of anatomical landmarks as the following:

- Forehead
- Eyebrow
- Eyelids: upper/lower
- Orbit
- Midface: nose, maxilla, upper lip, nasolabial folds, zygoma
- Lower face: lower lip, mandible, oral mucosa (buccal mucosa, upper lip sulcus, lower lip sulcus)

2.1 Methods of facial reconstruction

Methods commonly applied for facial resurfacing can be categorized as the followings:

- Tissue expansion
- Resection of tumor
- Repair with resurfacing
- Repair of multilayer defect
- Repair for functional purpose
- Recontouring with tissue restoration

Selection of method for facial resurfacing depends on location, etiology, functional and aesthetic considerations on each specific individual demands.

In this chapter, many kinds of situations for facial resurfacing are to be presented, with discussions explicitly depicted for each strategic approach.

3. Case presentations

1. Resurfacing with tissue expansion

    The patient sustained avulsion injury of right side forehead, resulting in a palm sized uneven unsightly scar. The right side temple and mid-forehead skin was then expanded by using 2 tissue expanders. Thereafter, the grafted area was removed with sufficient expansion of the forehead skin, which brought about much improved esthetic result (**Figure 1**).

2. Tissue expansion at grafted skin for auricular reconstruction.

    This 18 y/o boy had a big AVM at left ear and temple, which was excised and the ear was 3/5 amputated and then skin grafted during his childhood.

    To reconstruct his left ear, a 70 ml tissue expander was placed underneath the grafted skin. With gradual expansion at grafted skin, implantation of a carved rib cartilage graft for recontouring of his left ear was accomplished (**Figure 2**).

3. Facial resurfacing with resection of underlying AVM (arteriovenous malformation) at parotid gland, where skin had been expanded with the growth of the AVM.

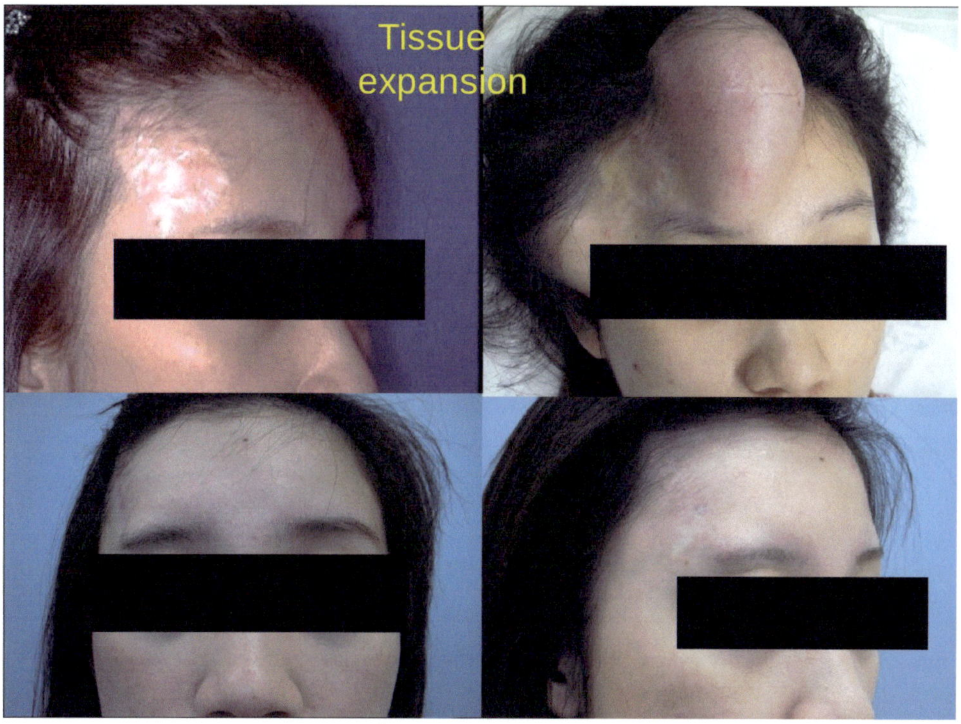

Figure 1.
Right forehead scar, treated with tissue expansion of neighboring flaps, excision of scar with primary closure. The remaining scar can be inconspicuous.

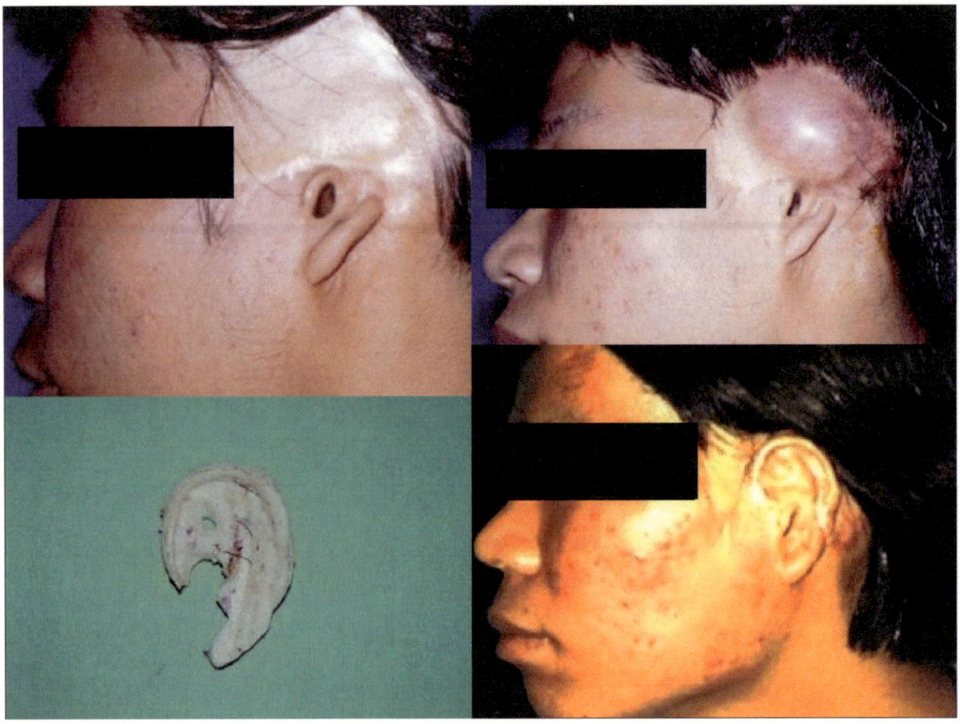

Figure 2.
Tissue expansion at grafted skin to accommodate a three dimensional carved auricular framework taken from costal cartilage block.

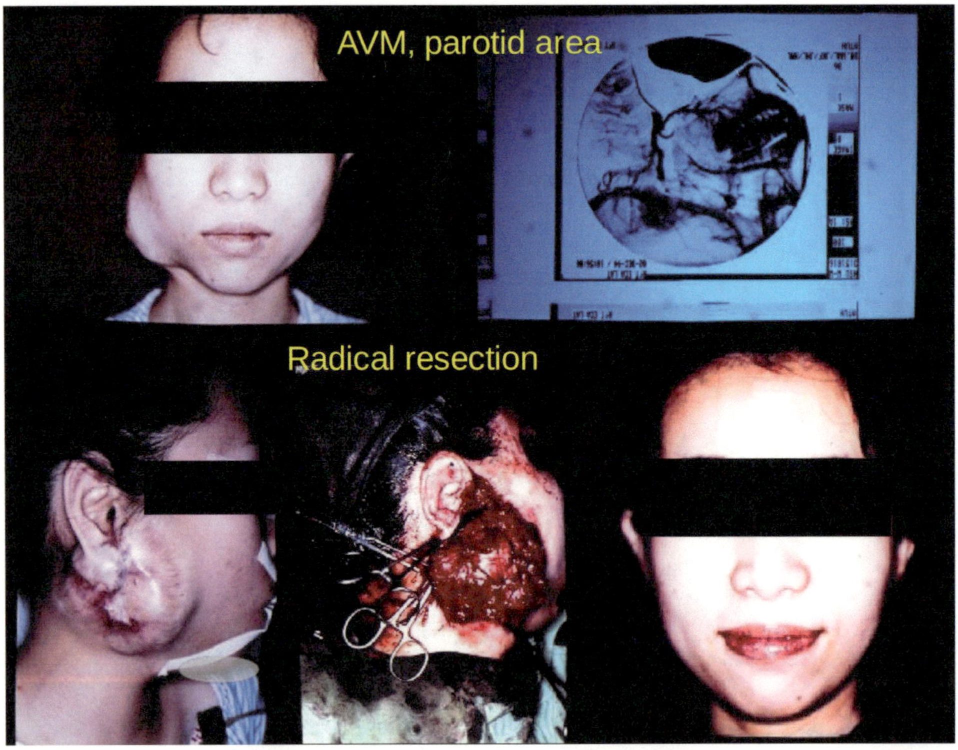

Figure 3.
With complete resection of the underlying AVM, the wound can be closed with pre-expanded skin flaps. The sunken right parotid area was filled with fat graft injection after 2 years. The patient regain satisfactory facial contour without facial asymmetry.

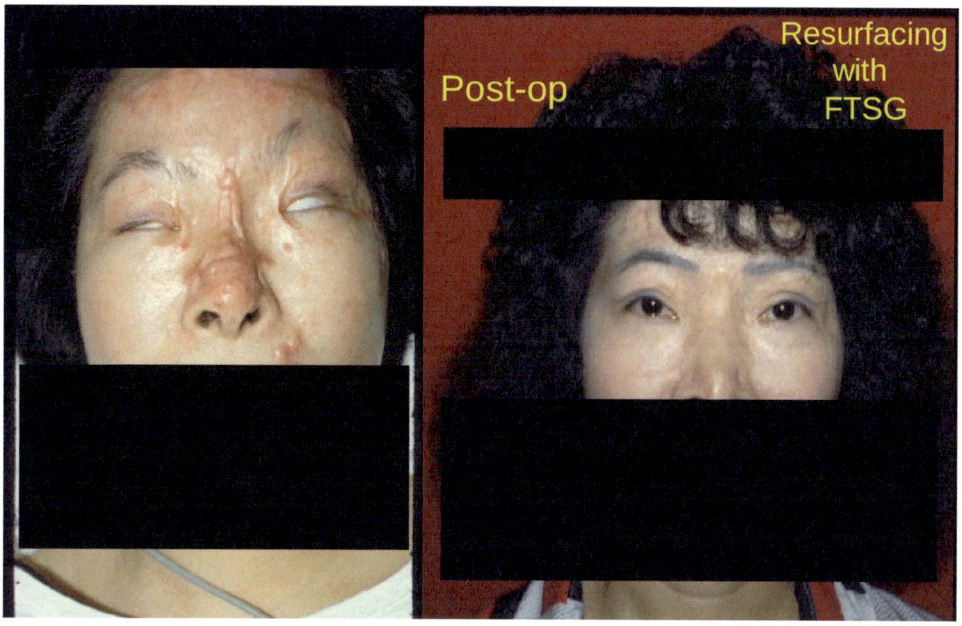

Figure 4.
Chemical burn facial contracture treated with: (1) resurfacing of nose with thick STSG; (2) releasing upper and lower eyelid scar contracture with FTSG; (3) resurfacing upper lip scar with FTSG; and (4) releasing forehead scar contracture to lower down the eyebrow and reconstruct left side forehead hairline with axial pattern scalp flap; followed by Kenacort A injection at remaining scars. Restoration of facial contour and symmetricity was obtained.

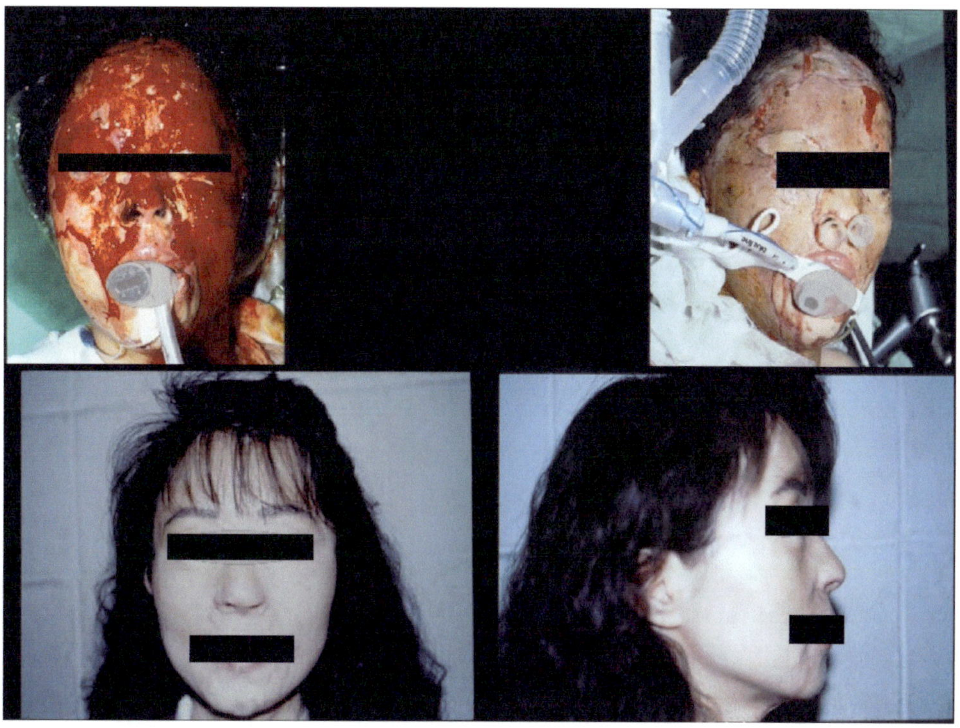

Figure 5.
This girl got assaulted with H_2SO_4, resulting in facial skin necrosis. Early tangential excision with early grafting following functional esthetic unit principle gave the girl a smooth, symmetric face.

4. The AVM was totally resected after arterial embolization, with complete preservation of the underlying facial nerve. After 2 years, fat grafting [9–11] was performed to fill the slightly sunken right parotid area. The patient regained satisfactory facial contour without facial asymmetry nor dynamic facial nerve dysfunction (**Figure 3**).

5. Facial scar contracture with ectropion, eyebrow asymmetry, nasal deformity and hypertrophic scarring. Anterior hairline reconstruction with hair-bearing scalp island flap, FTSG of bilateral upper and lower eyelids after release of scar contracture, thick STSG at nose and FTSG at upper lip after excision of hypertrophic scar were performed. The patient regained a smooth and symmetric face (**Figure 4**).

6. Major facial resurfacing with functional aesthetic unit concept and eyebrow scalp grafting (**Figure 5**) as primary treatment of a severe chemical burn patient (**Figure 5**).

7. Orbital reconstruction with free dorsalis pedis flap, conchal chondrocutaneous grafts, fat grafting, eyelash grafting with composite scalp graft (**Figure 6**).

   Expansion of orbital socket dimension with chondrocutaneous composite graft. Correction of enophthalmos with fat grafting and accommodation of an appropriate size of eye prosthesis, lateral canthopexy, creation of supratarsal fold, strip hair composite graft for eyelash followed.

8. The patient suffers from radiation necrosis of palate, resulting in a sizable palatal defect and scar contracture of soft palate and uvula.

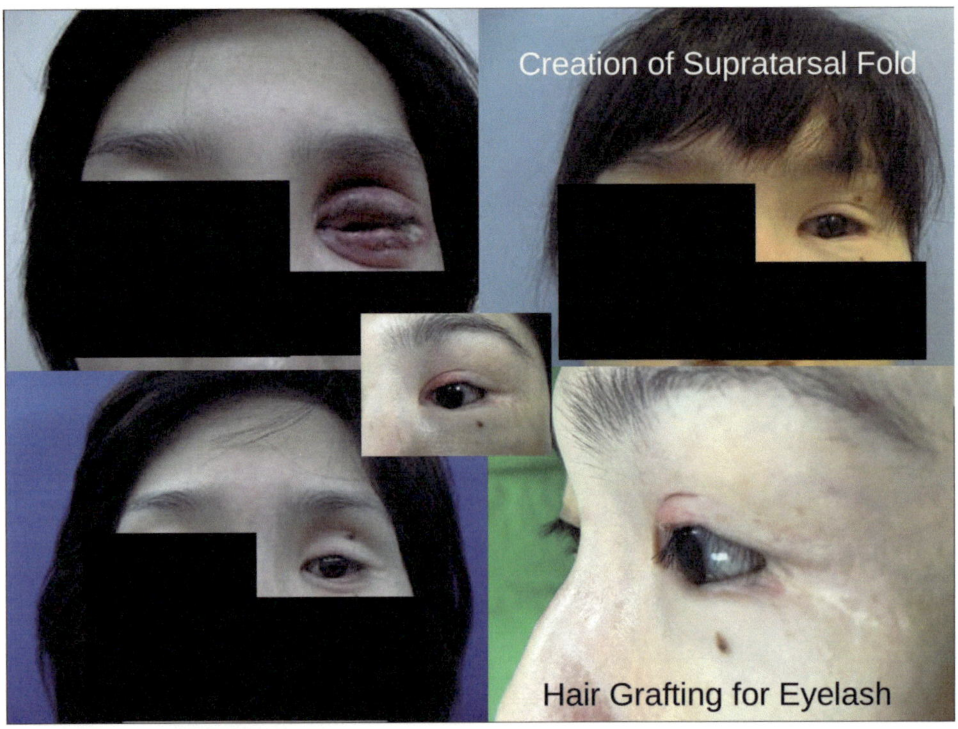

Figure 6.
Reconstruction of left orbital socket lining with dorsalis pedis free flap.

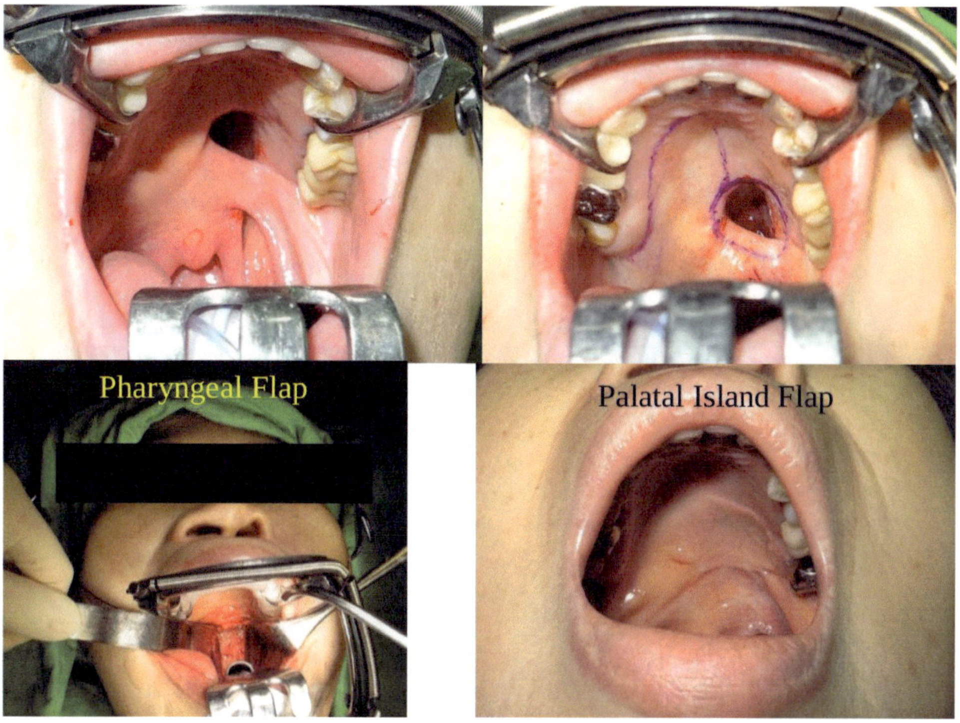

Figure 7.
(a) Radiation necrosis of hard palate and soft palate. (b) Right palatal flap was employed to repair the big oronasal fistula. (c) Pharyngeal flap was employed to hold the shortened uvula in order to ameliorate nasopharyngeal insufficiency.

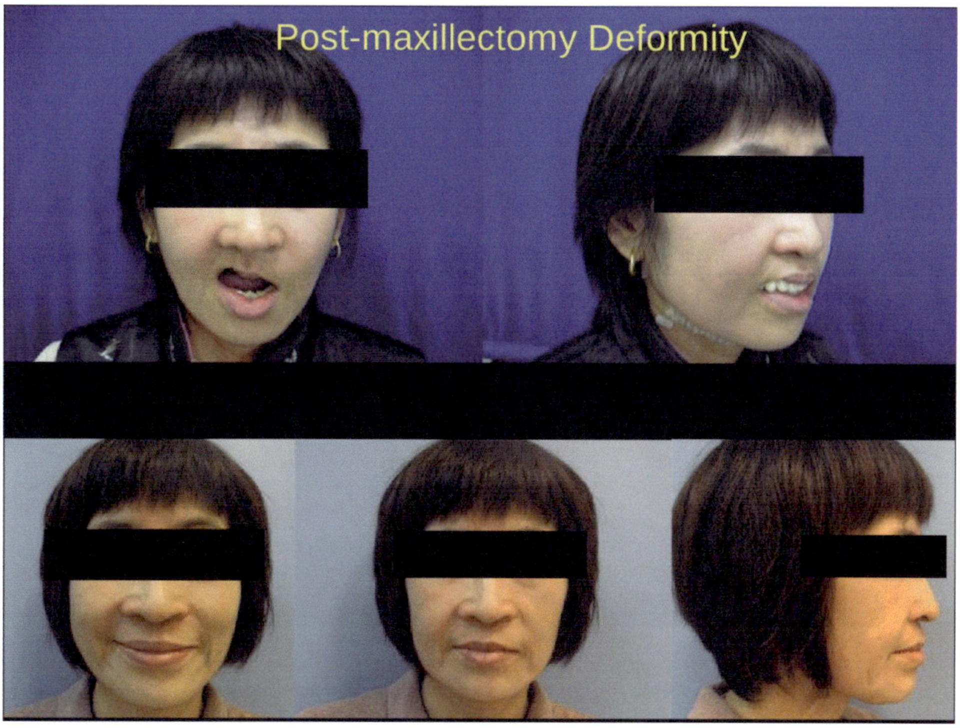

Figure 8.
Significant deformity after right maxillectomy for cancer.

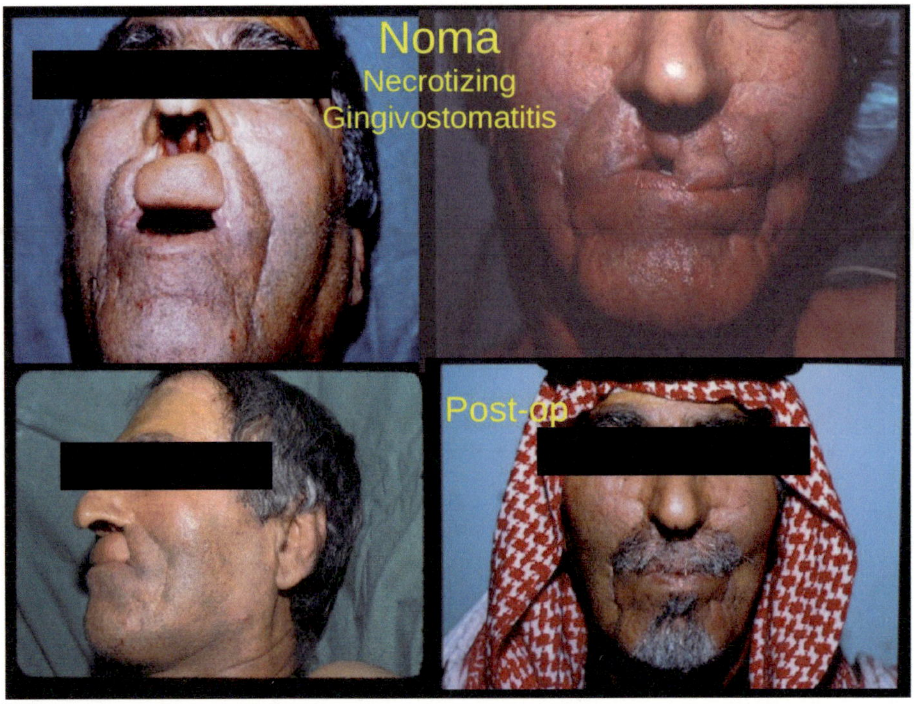

Figure 9.
This 57 y/o patient lost his upper lip, nasal base, and columella due to necrotizing gingivostomatitis. He had ever received upper lip reconstruction with forehead flap; however, the result was disappointing.

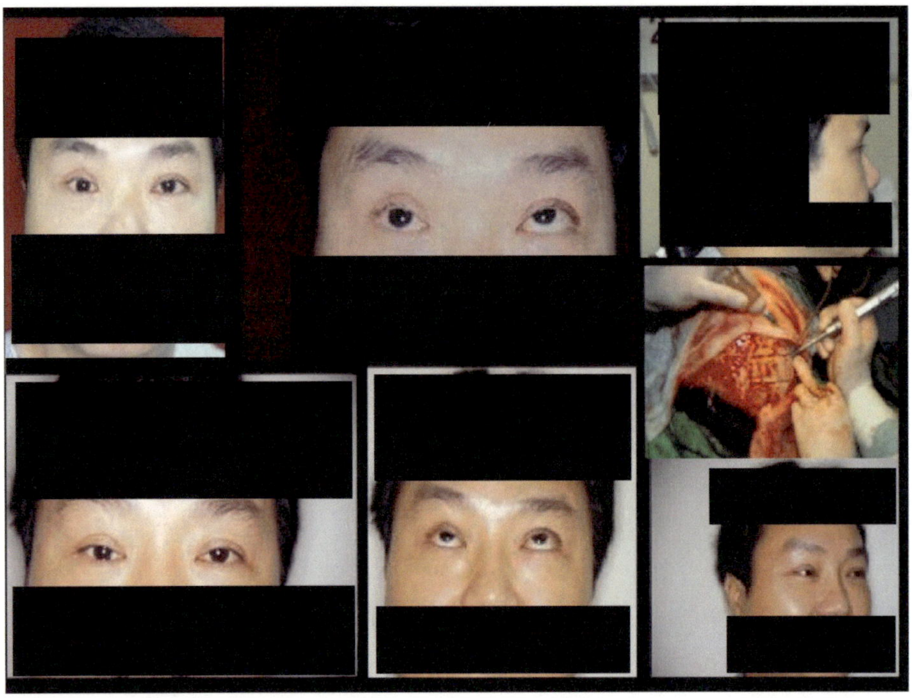

Figure 10.
Upper row: This patient got a panfacial fracture after a bad trauma. Diplopia owing to right orbital floor blow out fracture with enophthalmos and ptosis, flattening of nose due to untreated LeFort I, II, III maxillary fracture and displacement bothered him. Right middle: Calvarial bone grafting taken from the outer table of parietal bone was used to correct flat nose and right orbital floor bone defect, diplopia and enophthalmos (lower row). The patient was happy with the result.

Palatal arterial island flap of the right side was employed to cover the big palatal defect, and nasopharyngeal insufficiency was corrected with the use of pharyngeal flap to hold the uvula [2]. After the reconstruction, the patient was able to regain an intelligible speech (**Figure 7a–c**).

9. Significant deformity after right maxillectomy for cancer.

   Full thickness skin graft for maxillary contracture after complete release of the intraoral contracture was employed for reconstruction, followed by fitting a proper right maxillary obturator and upper denture (**Figure 8**).

   Full thickness skin graft for maxillary contracture after complete release of the intraoral contracture was employed for reconstruction, botox injection to lessen the activity of levator labii superioris, add volume to right side upper lip with hyaluronic acid, followed by fitting a proper right maxillary obturator and upper denture. The patient was happy to resume to a near normal appearance.

10. Reconstruction of complex upper lip, nasal floor and columella defect.

   The upper lip (**Figure 9**) flap was turned up to reconstruct the columella and nasal base, then Abbe flap from mid-lower lip was employed to reconstruct the

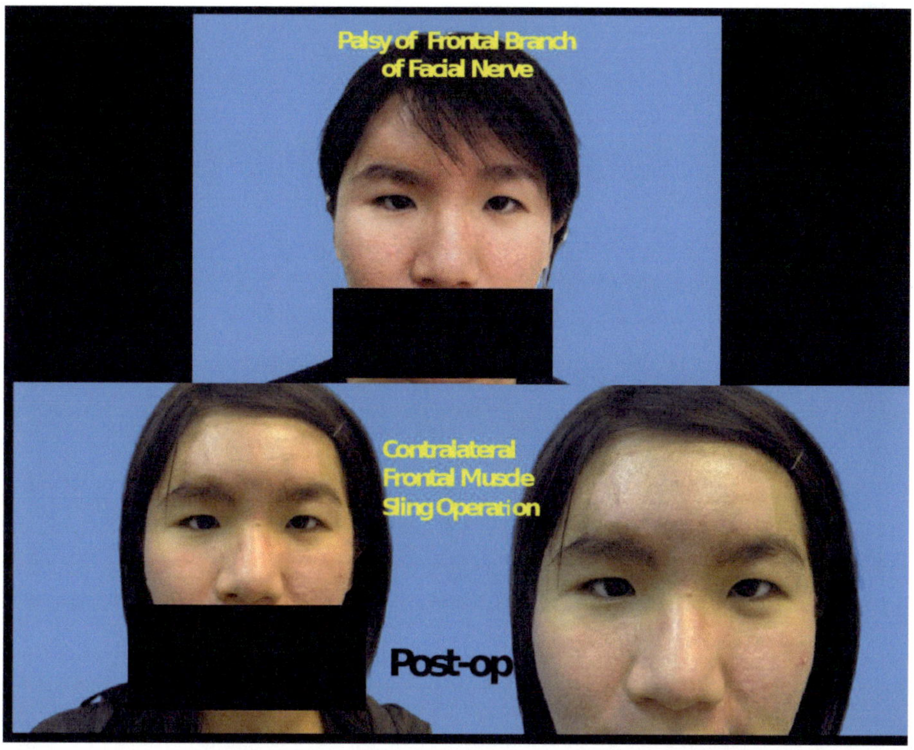

Figure 11.
This girl was a victim of train crash, resulting in avulsion laceration of right frontal area with frontal branch of facial nerve avulsion as well as zygomatic-orbital fracture displacement. She sustained palsy of right frontal branch facial nerve 8 months after operation, with asymmetry of right upper eyelid and eyebrow. Sling operation was employed with medial strip of frontal myoperiosteal flap to bring right eyebrow up to the right position. Upper row: pre-op; lower row: post-op.

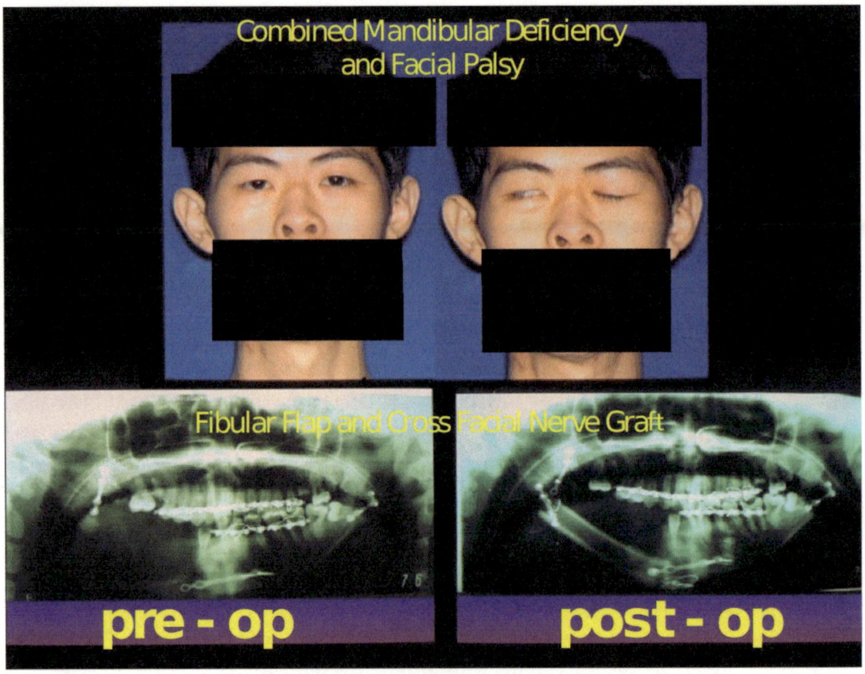

(a)

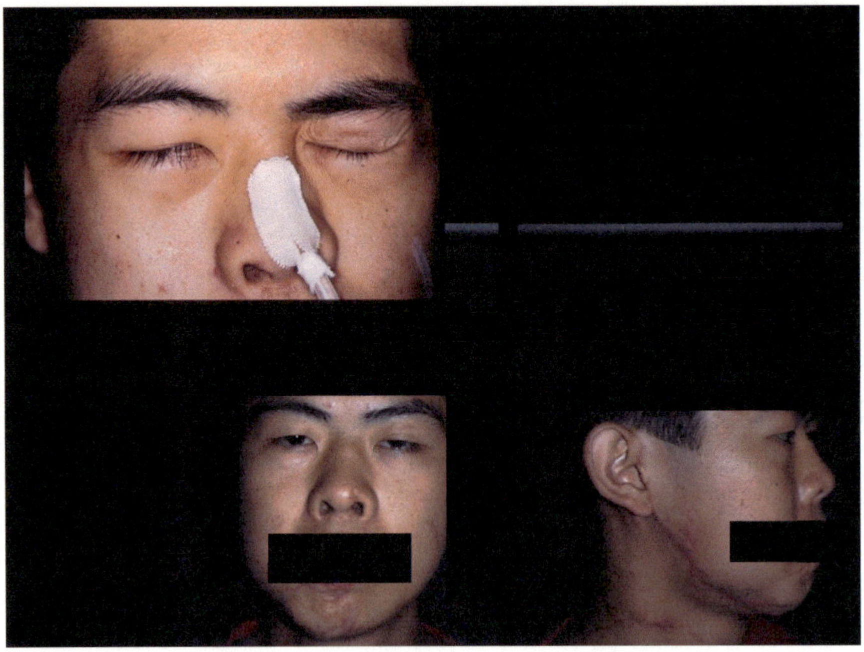

(b)

Figure 12.
(a) This 18 y/o boy was hit by a fallen wall during work, which resulted in compound comminuted fracture of right mandibular body, as well as right facial palsy and glossopharyngeal nerve palsy. Plating of right mandible was not successful, he was left with right mandibular defect and right facial palsy. He was referred to us 3 months later; then, we did free vascularized fibula mandibular reconstruction with concomitant cross facial nerve grafting at the same operation. After 3 months, the patient regained facial nerve function with good right mandibular contour. (b) Three months after free vascularized fibula mandibular reconstruction with concomitant cross facial nerve grafting at the same operation, the patient regained facial nerve function with good right mandibular contour.

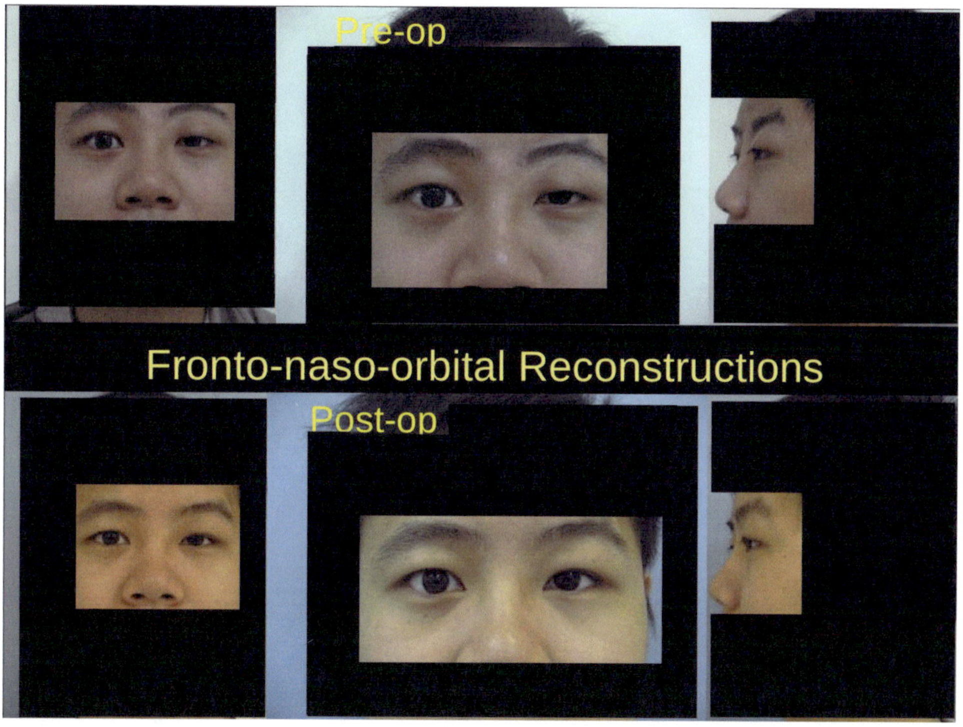

Figure 13.
This young man had a bad traffic accident, resulted in a frontonasal bone defect and left blepharoptosis (upper row). Reconstruction was accomplished with 3D CT reformation of the implant that is exactly the bony defect and contour of the defect, followed by correction of blepharoptosis (lower row).

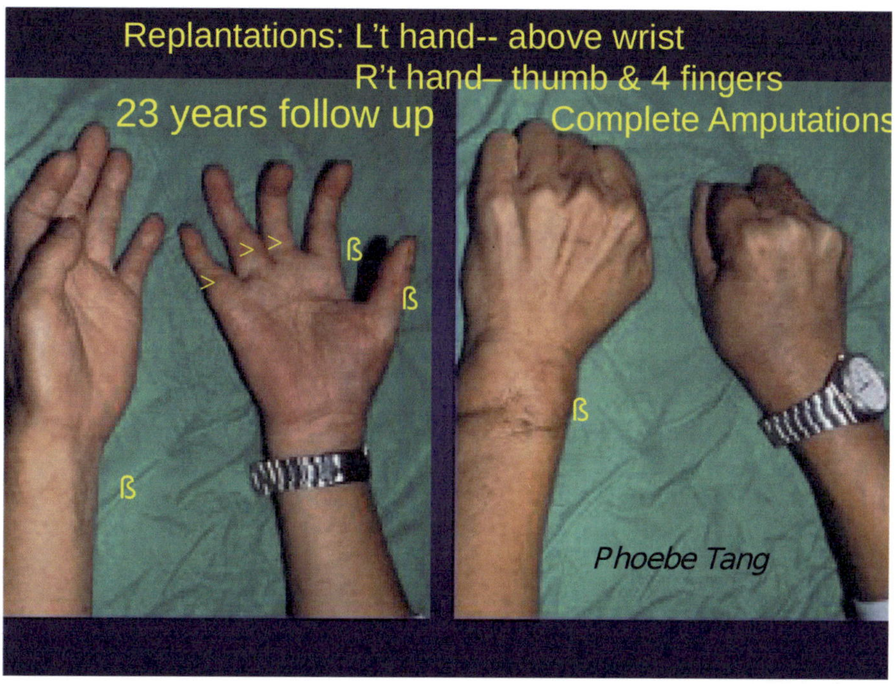

Figure 14.
This 30 y/o patient had his left forearm completely severed, and his right hand thumb and 4 fingers entirely cut by a machine. The amputated parts were completely replanted without any loss at all. The photo was taken 17 years later.

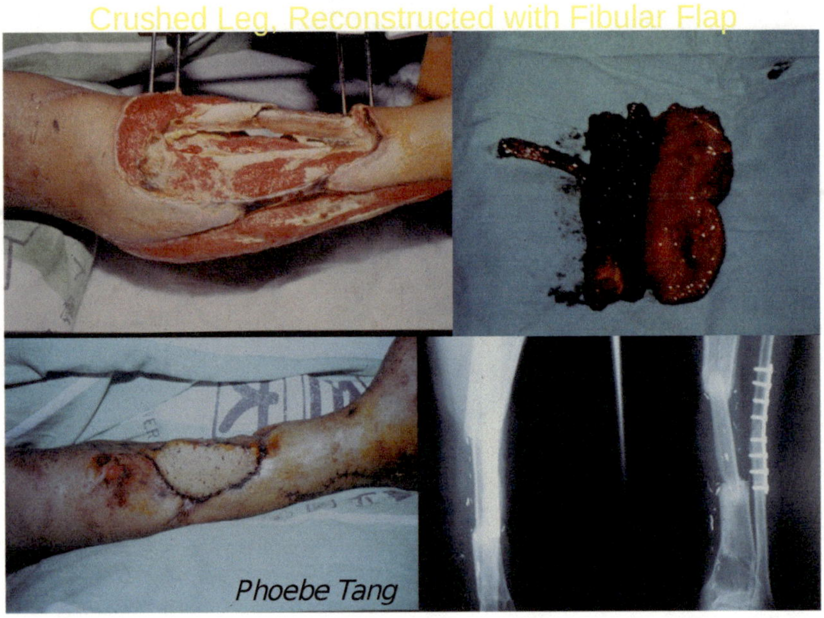

Figure 15.
This 26 y/o young man had his left leg run over by a high speed car at the superhighway. After serial debridement, the compound comminuted wound showed exposure of a long segment of tibia with denuded, devitalized bone with osteomyelitis. He was announced to receive above knee amputation, then he visited our service and was transferred for limb preserving surgery. The reconstruction was accomplished with plating of fractured fibula for stabilization, and concomitant debridement, resection of dried, infected bone, followed by harvesting contralateral fibula osteoseptocutaneous free flap to re-established the left tibia segmental continuity with artery and veins anastomosed at left posterior tibial artery and veins. The patient resumed walking 3 months after the operation, the vascularized fibula hypertrophied after weight bearing.

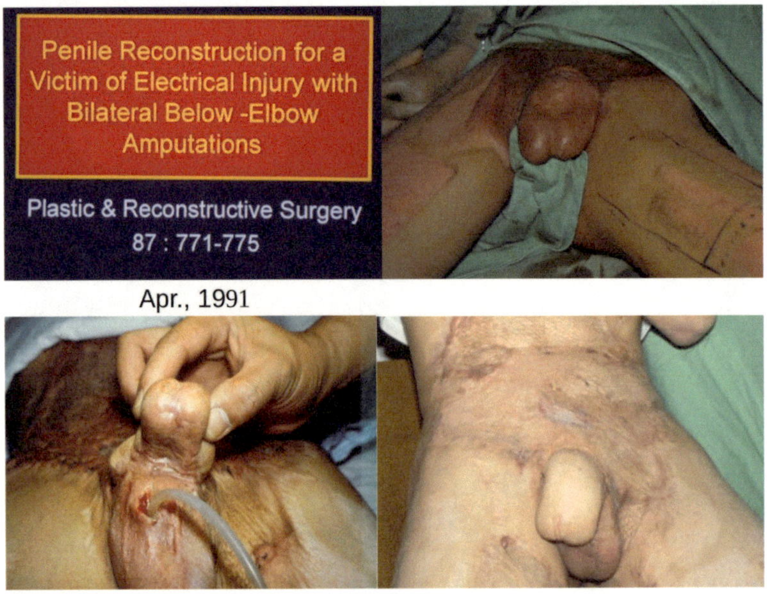

Figure 16.
This 18 y/o young man got a bad electrical injury, resulted in bilateral below elbow amputation and loss of penis, painful hypertrophic scars at entire abdomen. A jumping flap was performed by another surgeon, however cannot get a satisfactory result. He was referred to our service, where resurfacing of the abdomen was performed first to completely release the scar contracture (courtesy of plastic and reconstructive surgery).

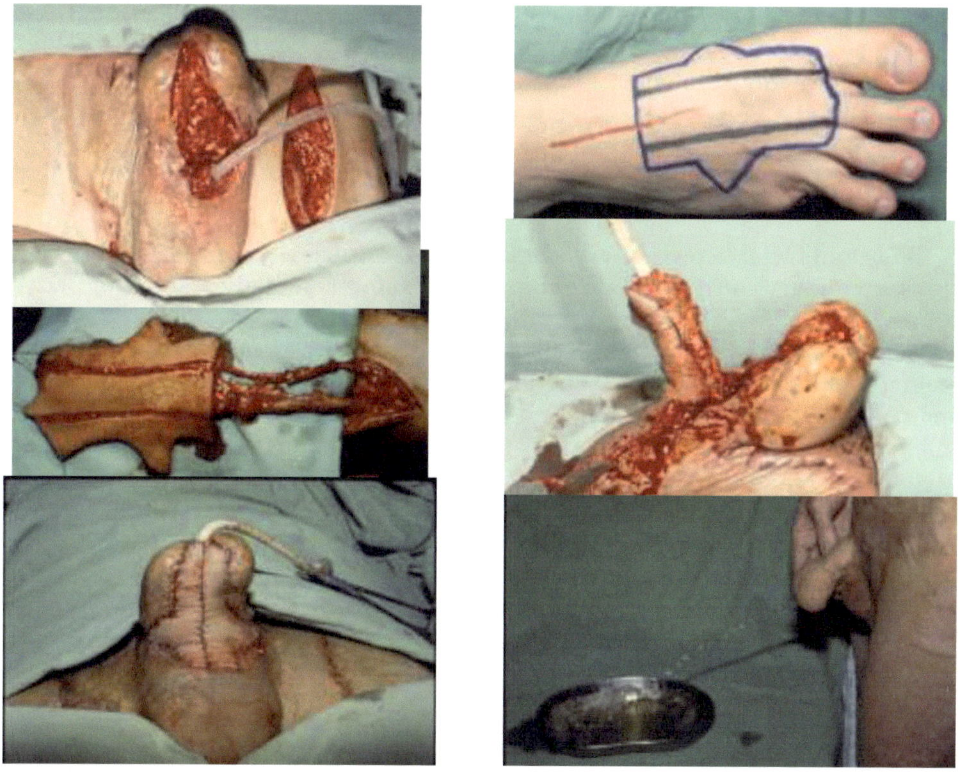

Figure 17.
Then reconstruction of the penile urethra was accomplished with a well-designed dorsalis pedis free flap, with simultaneous release of scar contracture in one operation. The wound healed uneventfully. This young man had been able to perform stand pissing. Two years later, a costal cartilage graft was employed to increase the rigidity of the reconstructed penis (courtesy of plastic and reconstructive surgery).

whole layer upper lip defect. The patient then regained a satisfactory facial appearance without noticeable disfigurement.

11. This patient got a panfacial fracture after a bad trauma (**Figure 10**). Diplopia owing to right orbital floor blow out fracture with enophthalmos and ptosis, flattening of nose due to untreated LeFort I, II, III maxillary fracture and displacement bothered him. Calvarial bone grafting taken from the outer table of parietal bone was used to correct flat nose and right orbital floor bone defect, diplopia and enophthalmos. The patient was happy with the result.

12. Palsy of the frontal branch of facial nerve (**Figure 11**).

13. Combined mandibular deficiency and facial palsy (**Figure 12a** and **b**).

14. Traffic accident, resulted in a frontonasal bone defect and left blepharoptosis (**Figure 13**).

15. Complete severance of left forearm; right thumb and four fingers (**Figure 14**).

    He had been able to take care of himself with good function and sensibility at both hands. He got a stable job, got married and raised children with a good family.

16. Crushed leg, reconstructed with fibula osteoseptocutaneous free flap (**Figure 15**).

17. Reconstruction of penile loss due to electrical injury (**Figures 16a** and **17**).

4. Discussion

Body and facial defect, injury, congenital deformities, status post-tumor excisions, secondary contractures are common encounters in daily practice of plastic surgeons.

In this chapter, we present miscellaneous kinds of measures employed for resurfacing, contour restoration and functional rehabilitation of the face, extremity, and body parts. Tissue expansion, tumor excision, skin grafting (split thickness/full thickness), composite graft, cartilage graft, hair composite graft are commonly used measures. Flap surgery should be elaborated in proper situations. Selection of proper tissue for reconstruction is of utmost importance.

The ailments that were cited and treated are as the followings:

Problems	Solutions
1. Forehead trauma, with facial disfigurement	Tissue expansion
2. s/p right auricle amputation with skin graft	Tissue expansion at grafted skin with implantation of carved rib cartilage graft for ear reconstruction
3. AVM at parotid area	Complete excision
4. Scar contracture at face with secondary	FTSG, thick STSG, scalp deformities, arterial skin island flap
5. Chemical burn facial defects	Early FTSG at functional esthetic units
6. Orbital reconstruction	Free dorsalis pedis flap, conchal chondrocutan eous grafts, fat graft, free dorsalis pedis flap, conchal chondrocutan eous grafts, fat graft, eyelash composite graft
7. Radiation necrosis of palate	Palatal island flap, pharyngeal flap
8. Maxillary defect, contracture	FTSG, upper denture with stent
9. Reconstruction of complex upper lip	Abbe flap nasal floor and columella defect
10. Panfacial fracture	Calvarial bone graft
11. Palsy of the frontal branch of facial nerve	Frontalis sling operation
12. Combined mandibular deficiency, facial palsy	Fibular flap; cross facial nerve graft
13. Frontonasal bone defect, left blepharoptosis	3D CT bone reformation
14. Complete severance of left forearm	Replantation right thumb and 4 fingers
15. Crushed leg with tibial defect	Fibula osteocutaneous free flap
16, 17. Penile loss due to electrical injury	Dorsalis pedis free flap

The flaps that we described and introduced in this chapter were as the followings: forehead flap, Abbe flap for upper lip reconstruction, cheek flap, nasolabial flap for nasal defects, greater palatine artery flap and pharyngeal flap for complex palatal defect, dorsalis pedis free flap for penile and urethal reconstruction, free fibular osteoseptocutaneous flap for reconstruction of composite bone and skin defect of the lower extremity.

5. Conclusion

Difficult reconstructions are not only challenging, but also formidable tasks in terms of anatomical restoration, functional rehabilitation and esthetic refinements. With deliberate planning, selection of proper measure and tissue for reconstruction, optimal results can always be achieved. Pursuing excellence in plastic surgery, bringing excellence to life has always been our ultimate goals.

Acknowledgements

The authors are indebted to Mr. Ming-Chieh Li for his help in editing this manuscript.

Author details

Shihheng Chen[1], Hung-Chi Chen[2] and Yueh-Bih Tang[3,4,5,6]*

1 Chang-Gung Memorial Hospital at Linko, New Taipei City, Taiwan

2 China Medical University Hospital, Taichung, Taiwan

3 Far-Eastern Memorial Hospital at Banqiao, New Taipei City, Taiwan

4 National Taiwan University Hospital, Taipei, Taiwan

5 Plastic Surgery Society of Taiwan, Taiwan

6 Aesthetic Surgery Society of Taiwan, Taiwan

*Address all correspondence to: phoebetang0103@gmail.com

References

[1] Rosen HM. Definitive surgical correction of vertical maxillary deficiency. Plastic and Reconstructive Surgery. 1990;**85**:215

[2] Rosen HM. Facial skeletal expansion: Treatment strategies and rationale. Plastic and Reconstructive Surgery. 1992;**89**:798

[3] Mordick TG 2nd, Larossa D, Whitaker L. Soft-tissue reconstruction of the face: A comparison of dermal fat grafting and vascularized tissue transfer. Annals of Plastic Surgery. 1992;**9**:390-396

[4] Siebert JW, Longaker MT. Secondary craniofacial management following skeletal correction in facial asymmetry. Application of microsurgical technique. Clinics in Plastic Surgery. 1997;**24**:447-458

[5] Siebert JW, Anson G, Longaker MT. Microsurgical correction of facial asymmetry in 60 consecutive cases. Plastic and Reconstructive Surgery. 1996;**97**:354-363

[6] Longaker MT, Siebert JW. Microsurgical correction of facial contour in congenital craniofacial malformations: The marriage of hard and soft tissue. Plastic and Reconstructive Surgery. 1996;**98**:942-950

[7] McCarthy J. Cutting C: Secondary deformities of cleft lip and palate. In: Georgiade NG, Riefkohl R, Barwick W, editors. Textbook of Plastic, Maxillofacial and Reconstructive Surgery. Baltimore: Williams & Wilkins; 1992. pp. 307-319

[8] Tang YB, Randall P. Reconstruction for complex upper lip, nasal base and columella defect. Plastic and Reconstructive Surgery. 1991;**87**:771-775

[9] Chen PR, Tang YB. Dorsalis pedis free flap for reconstruction of full thickness cheek defect in buccal cancer—Case report. Journal of Otolaryngological Society R.O.C. 1992;**27**:401

[10] Tang YB. Major mandibular reconstruction with vascularized bone grafts, indications and selection of donor tissue. Microsurgery;**15**:227

[11] Chen SH, Chen HK, Horng SY, Yeong EK, Tang YB. Reconstruction for osteoradionecrosis of the mandible: Superiority of free iliac bone flap to fibula flap in terms of postoperative infection and healing. Annals of Plastic Surgery. 2014;**73**(Suppl 1):S18-S26